PRIMARY HEALTH CARE AND COMPLEMENTARY AND INTEGRATIVE MEDICINE

PRACTICE AND RESEARCH

PRIMARY HEALTH CARE AND COMPLEMENTARY AND INTEGRATIVE MEDICINE

PRACTICE AND RESEARCH

Editors

Jon Adams
University of Technology Sydney, Australia

Parker Magin
University of Newcastle, Australia

Alex Broom
The University of Queensland, Australia

Imperial College Press

ICP

Published by

Imperial College Press
57 Shelton Street
Covent Garden
London WC2H 9HE

Distributed by

World Scientific Publishing Co. Pte. Ltd.
5 Toh Tuck Link, Singapore 596224
USA office: 27 Warren Street, Suite 401-402, Hackensack, NJ 07601
UK office: 57 Shelton Street, Covent Garden, London WC2H 9HE

Library of Congress Cataloging-in-Publication Data
Primary health care and complementary and integrative medicine : practice and research / edited by
Jon Adams.
    p. ; cm.
    Includes bibliographical references and index.
    ISBN 978-1-84816-977-7 (hardcover : alk. paper)
    I. Adams, Jon, 1971–
    [DNLM: 1. Integrative Medicine--methods. 2. Complementary Therapies.
3. Primary Health Care. WB 113]

    616--dc23
                                    2012048471

British Library Cataloguing-in-Publication Data
A catalogue record for this book is available from the British Library.

Typeset by Stallion Press
Email: enquiries@stallionpress.com

Printed in Singapore by World Scientific Printers.

Contents

List of Figures   vii

List of Tables   ix

Notes on Contributors   xi

Acknowledgements   xxiii

Introduction   1

Part One   **Patients, Illness and Disease: CIM Use
                and its Context in Primary Health Care**   9

Chapter 1   Primary Health Care, Complementary
                and Alternative Medicine and Women's Health:
                A Focus upon Menopause   11
                Amie Steel, Jane Frawley, Jon Adams,
                David Sibbritt, and Alex Broom

Chapter 2   Complementary and Integrative Medicine, Aging
                and Chronic Illness: Towards an Interprofessional
                Approach in Primary Health Care   35
                Kevin D. Willison, Sally Lindsay, Marissa Taylor,
                Harold Schroeder, and Gavin J. Andrews

Chapter 3   Complementary and Alternative Medicine
                and Skin Disease in General Practice   51
                Parker Magin and Jon Adams

Part Two   **Practitioners and the Professional CIM Interface** 71

Chapter 4   Naturopaths: Their Role in Primary
                Health Care Delivery   73
                Jon Wardle and Jon Adams

Chapter 5   Linking Complementary and Alternative Medicine,
             Traditional Medicine and Primary Health Care:
             The Role of Local Health Traditions in Promoting
             Health Security   93
             Daniel Hollenberg and Maria Costanza Torri

Chapter 6   Examining the Relationship between
             Complementary and Integrative Medicine
             and Rural General Practice: A Focus upon
             Health Services Research   115
             Jon Wardle, Jon Adams, Alex Broom,
             and David Sibbritt

Chapter 7   (Just) Who is the Expert? The Ambiguity of
             Expertise in Over-the-Counter CAM Purchasing:
             An Ethnographic Study of UK Community
             Pharmacies and Health Shops   133
             Helen Cramer, Lesley Wye,
             Marjorie Weiss, and Ali Shaw

**Part Three   Conceptualising Integrative Medicine in Primary
             Health Care: Experience and Challenges   155**

Chapter 8   Integrating Complementary Medicine
             in Primary Health Care as a Response
             to Contemporary Challenges: A Focus upon
             Effectiveness Gaps and Self-Care   157
             David Peters

Chapter 9   Exploring a Model of Integrative Medicine:
             A Case Study in Swedish Primary Health Care   181
             Tobias Sundberg

Chapter 10   Integration in Primary Health Care: A Focus
             upon Practice and Education and the Importance
             of a Critical Social Science Perspective   203
             Jon Adams, Daniel Hollenberg, Alex Broom,
             Amie Steel, David Sibbritt, and Chi-Wai Lui

Index   229

List of Figures

Figure 2.1   Dialectical strategies to enhance primary health
             care (PHC) for the aged. Legend: PHC = primary
             health care; CDM = chronic disease management;
             CAM = complementary and alternative medicine;
             IPE/IPC = interprofessional education,
             interprofessional collaboration   36

Figure 9.1   An outline of the qualitative procedures
             and analyses developing the IM model
             (Sundberg *et al.*, 2007)   183

Figure 9.2   The IM model and the IM care process illustrated
             as a clinical case management flowchart:
             (1) The patient with subacute to chronic non-specific
             LBP/NP consults the gatekeeping general practitioner
             at the primary care unit, (2) The general practitioner
             develops a conventional care treatment plan in
             dialogue with the patient, (3) The patient goes through
             the conventional care process, i.e., "treatment
             as usual", (4) Should CTs be considered appropriate,
             these are integrated into the treatment plan by way
             of a consensus case conference with the IM provider
             team, (5) The patient receives CTs as an integrated part
             of the treatment plan, i.e., the integrative care process
             is initiated, (6) When the treatment plan is completed
             the case management is finished. Please note that for
             the current research project the patients were assigned
             by randomisation and integrative care was only
             delivered for up to 12 weeks. PC Unit = primary
             care unit (Sundberg *et al.*, 2007)   187

List of Tables

Table 1.1   Consultations with alternative health
             practitioners in the previous 12 months   18
Table 1.2   Self-prescribed treatments used in the previous
             12 months   19
Table 1.3   Attitudes towards alternative medicine
             and doctors   20
Table 1.4   Access to and satisfaction with general
             practitioners   21

Table 7.1   Key characteristics of each of the six study sites   139

Table 7.2   Comparison of key characteristics
             of the six study sites   146

Table 8.1   How the Self-Care Library codes the evidence,
             safety and cost   169
Table 8.2   An example of the way the Self-Care Library
             categorises information   170

Notes on Contributors

Jon Adams is Professor of Public Health at the Faculty of Health, University of Technology Sydney, Australia, where he leads a national team of 12 CAM researchers and he holds a prestigious National Health and Medical Research Council (NHMRC) Career Development Fellowship (the only one to be focused upon CAM research). Jon is Executive Director of the Network of Researchers in the Public Health of Complementary and Alternative Medicine (NORPHCAM) www.nor-phcam.org and a Senior Fellow of the International Brisbane Initiative, Department of Primary Health Care, University of Oxford. Jon is also National Convenor of the 'Evidence, Research and Policy in Complementary Medicine' Special Interest Group at the Public Health Association of Australia (PHAA), Associate Editor for the peer-reviewed journals *Complementary Therapies in Medicine*, *Journal of Acupuncture and Meridian Studies*, and *BMC Complementary and Alternative Medicine* as well as Regional Co-Editor for the *European Journal of Integrative Medicine*. Jon has authored over 170 peer-reviewed publications since 2001 and he is Editor/Co-Editor of six international health research books including Editor-in-Chief of *Traditional, Complementary and Alternative Medicine: An International Reader* (Palgrave Macmillan, 2012), *Mainstreaming Complementary and Alternative Medicine: Studies in Social Context* (Routledge, 2003), *Complementary and Alternative Medicine in Nursing and Midwifery: Towards a Critical Social Science* (Routledge, 2007), *Researching Complementary and Alternative Medicine* (Routledge. 2006), and *Evidence-Based Healthcare in Context: Critical Social Science Perspectives* (Ashgate, 2011). Jon's current research programmes, attracting competitive external funding from NHMRC, ARC and PHCRED, span a wide range of interests including developing the public health perspective of TCIM, examining CAM in relation to primary health care, rural health, women's health, chronic illness, and the wider context of self-care, as well as exploring the potential of traditional medicine in addressing contemporary global health issues.

Gavin J. Andrews is a professor at McMaster University, Canada. Gavin was the inaugural Chair of the Department of Health, Aging and Society from 2006–2011. A health geographer and predominantly qualitative researcher, Gavin's wide-ranging interests include the dynamics between space/place and complementary medicine, aging, nursing, specific phobias, fitness, health histories, popular music, and primary health care. Much of Gavin's work is positional and considers the development, state-of-the-art, and future of his sub-discipline. Gavin's particular interests in complementary medicine include small business entrepreneurship, visualization practices, and the use of music as an everyday practice for well-being. Gavin has published 120 journal articles and book chapters, three journal special editions (two in *Social Science & Medicine,* 2007 & 2009), and three books: *Aging and Place: Perspectives, Policy, Practice* (Routledge, 2006), *The Sociology of Aging: A Reader* (Rawat, 2009), and *Primary Health Care: People, Practice, Place* (Ashgate, 2008). Gavin is currently preparing another edited book for Ashgate called *Medicinal Melodies: Places of Health and Wellbeing in Popular Music* (expected 2013).

Alex Broom is Associate Professor of Sociology and Australia Research Council Future Fellow at the School of Social Science, The University of Queensland, Australia. Alex specializes in the sociology of traditional, complementary, and alternative medicine (TCAM) and the sociology of cancer and end-of-life care and he has led sociological studies of TCAM in Australia, the UK, Brazil, India, Pakistan and Sri Lanka. Alex is currently leading a cross-cultural comparative study of medical pluralism in Australia, India, and Brazil and a longitudinal qualitative study of end-of-life care in Australia. Recent co-authored and co-edited books include: *Traditional, Complementary and Alternative Medicine and Cancer Care* (Routledge, 2007), *Therapeutic Pluralism* (Routledge, 2008), *Men's Health: Body, Identity and Social Context* (Wiley-Blackwell, 2009), *Health, Culture and Religion in South Asia* (Routledge, 2011), and *Evidence-Based Healthcare in Context: Critical Social Science*

Perspectives (Ashgate, 2011). Alex is a Visiting Professor at Jawaharlal Nehru University, India and Brunel University, UK, and he is an Honorary Associate Professor at the University of Sydney, Australia. Alex is also Director of Social Science Research for the Network of Researchers in the Public Health of CAM (www.norphcam.org).

Helen Cramer is a NIHR School for Primary Care Research Postdoctoral Research Fellow in the Centre for Academic Primary Care, School of Social and Community Medicine, University of Bristol, UK. She has a background in Medical and Social Anthropology and continues to use anthropological perspectives, specializing in qualitative research, applied research and research which uses an ethnographic methodology. Helen has a wide range of interests in health, self-care, gender, and health care services, spanning both primary and secondary care. Helen's current research projects focus mainly in the clinical areas of mental health and cardiovascular disease including the use of group therapy formats for depression and anxiety, masculinity, help seeking, depression and anxiety, the inter-relationship between depression, anxiety and cardiovascular disease, angina and the use of medical technologies in diagnosis, unplanned admissions for heart failure, and inter-hospital differences in the care and outcomes of patients with heart attacks. Helen's PhD was based in the Department of Urban Studies at Glasgow University, UK, where she researched the ethnography of gender and homelessness.

Jane Frawley is a PhD candidate at the Faculty of Health, University of Technology Sydney, Australia. She also holds a Bachelor of Complementary Medicine from Charles Sturt University, Australia, and a Master of Clinical Science from Southern Cross University, Australia. Jane served as an Examiner and Board Director for the National Herbalists Association of Australia (NHAA) for many years and is currently Chair of a subcommittee for the Australian Register of Naturopaths and Herbalists (ARONAH), examining appropriate education standards for naturopaths and herbalists in Australia. Jane has published numerous peer-reviewed articles on complementary medicine and is an Editorial Board Member of the *Australian Journal of Medical Herbalism.* Jane has also authored chapters for numerous books including *Clinical Naturopathic Medicine*

(Churchill Livingstone, 2012), *Clinical Naturopathy: An Evidence-Based Guide to Practice* (Churchill Livingstone, 2010) and *Herbs and Natural Supplements: An Evidence-Based Guide* (Churchill Livingstone, 2010).

Ali Heawood (née Shaw) is a Senior Research Fellow in the Centre for Academic Primary Care, University of Bristol, UK, where she specializes in qualitative research applied to a range of health care issues. She previously completed a Department of Health funded Postdoctoral Fellowship award on patients' experiences of complementary therapy use (2003–2006). This led to a series of complementary therapy related projects over the following years, including a study of advice-giving for over-the-counter complementary health care products in pharmacies and health shops. Other complementary therapy studies she has been involved in include a study of patient and parent decision-making about complementary therapies for asthma, homeopathy as an adjunct to usual care for children with asthma, male cancer patients' complementary therapy use, holistic care for patients with cancer, and family beliefs and decision-making about complementary therapies. She has published findings from her complementary therapy research in journals such as *Journal of Alternative and Complementary Medicine, European Journal of Integrative Medicine, Health and Social Care in the Community, Health Expectations, BMC Health Services Research*, and *BMC Complementary and Alternative Medicine*. More broadly, her interests include patient experiences of health and illness, patient decision-making, patient-practitioner communication, mental health in the primary care context, how health care services are organized and delivered, the use of qualitative methods within and alongside randomized trials, and the synthesis of qualitative research using methods such as meta-ethnography.

Daniel Hollenberg is Research Associate with the Office of Health Policy, Royal College of Physicians and Surgeons of Canada, Ottawa, Canada. He received his doctorate in Community Health from the University of Toronto, Canada, where he conducted a pioneering study of integrative medicine settings in Canada. His postdoctoral work at McMaster University and the University of Ottawa explored the introduction of CAM in Canadian hospital settings with comparative research in Shanghai, China. With a strong background in Medical Anthropology and Medical Sociology, Daniel maintains broad research interests related to integrative medicine including clinics and hospital settings, interprofessional education and collaboration amongst CAM and bio-medical professions, traditional medicine, and international/global health. Daniel has published numerous peer-reviewed articles and book chapters related to these research areas. Currently, he is leading the first in-depth study of traditional, complementary and alternative medicine use in rural/remote areas of Ontario, Canada, including First Nations/Aboriginal healing.

Sally Lindsay is a scientist at the Bloorview Research Institute, Holland Bloorview Kids Rehabilitation Hospital, Toronto, Canada. She is also an Associate Professor in the Departments of Occupational Science & Occupational Therapy and the Graduate Department of Rehabilitation Sciences, University of Toronto, Canada. Her work primarily focuses on social inclusion plus participation, health, and well-being of children and youth with disabilities.

Chi-Wai Lui is a lecturer in the School of Population Health at the University of Queensland, Australia. He is a member of the Network of Researchers in the Public Health of Complementary and Alternative Medicine (NORPHCAM, http://www.norphcam.org/) and the "Evidence, Research and Policy in Complementary Medicine" Special Interest Group at the Public Health Association of Australia. Chi-Wai is a soci-ologist by training and has actively engaged in a broad range of research projects on issues of health service use, chronic illness management, ageing, globalization and migrant settlement. Over the past three years he has worked as Project Manager on a large research project funded by the National Health and Medical Research Council investigating the use of complementary and alternative medicine among rural and urban women in Australia. Chi-Wai has authored 27 peer-reviewed publications in the last four years and is a regular reviewer of international journals including *Ageing & Society*, *BMC Complementary and Alternative Medicine*, *Complementary Therapies in Medicine*, and the *Australasian Journal on Ageing*.

Parker Magin is a general practitioner and Senior Lecturer and Director of the Primary Health Care Research, Evaluation and Development Program, Discipline of General Practice, at the University of Newcastle, Australia, and a medical educator at General Practice Training Valley to Coast, Newcastle, Australia. Parker is also a key collaborator with the Network of Researchers in the Public Health of Complementary and Alternative Medicine (NORPHCAM), an affiliated researcher with the Brain and Mental Health Program, Hunter Medical Research Institute and a member of the Royal Australian College of General Practitioners Standing Committee — Research. Parker has authored over 50 peer-reviewed publications in the last six years. A primary research interest has been skin disease in general practice, including the use of CAM therapies for skin diseases. Other areas of research interest are occupational violence in general practice, stroke and cerebral transient ischaemic attacks, and the clinical experiences of general practice vocational trainees.

David Peters is Professor of Integrated Healthcare and Clinical Director, School of Integrated Health, University of Westminster, UK. David qualified in medicine in 1972 and studied homeopathy at Glasgow Homeopathic Hospital in the mid-1970s, and explored it further in an anthroposophical community in Scotland where he lived for three years before returning to London to train in mainstream family medicine in 1979. The family practice in Uxbridge where David trained with Dr John English was one of first to use complementary medicine in the NHS. In the early 1980s David began working with Patrick Pietroni, first teaching medical students about family medicine at St Mary's Medical School, UK, and subsequently as a postgraduate GP trainer. In the mid-1980s David helped establish the British Holistic Medical Association (BHMA) and was Chair of the BHMA intermittently for many years until 2010. In 1987, David joined the Marylebone Health Centre (MHC) a ground-breaking Central London NHS GP unit established by Professor Patrick Pietroni. A substantial grant from the Waites Foundation enabled MHC's multidisciplinary team to explore new approaches to inner-city primary health care. From 1990 until 2005 David directed the centre's complementary therapies programme, which was described in *Integrating Complementary Therapies in Primary Care* (Harcourt, Edinburgh, 2002). David has co-authored and edited five books on integrated health care and led a series of projects concerned with implementing and evaluating complementary therapies in mainstream settings. One recent project explored the use of acupuncture and osteopathy for low back pain in a family practice centre (http://www. biomedcentral.com/1471–2296/12/49); another developed area-wide access to acupuncture and stress reduction for people with long-term low back pain. David edits the *Journal of Holistic Healthcare* (http://www. bhma.org/pages/journal.php) and he is a director of the recently formed College of Medicine which aims to encourage more patient-centred and values-based approaches in health care. David's clinical work as a mus-culo-skeletal physician has been greatly enriched by the perspectives of osteopathy and acupuncture and somatically oriented psychotherapy, as well as by his own exploration of the relaxation response, yoga, and medi-tation. David's research interests include the role of non-pharmaceutical treatments in mainstream medicine and self-care — particularly in long-term conditions — as well as the implementation of integrative practice and the education of more integrated practitioners.

Harold Schroeder is a senior level management consultant and strategic project manager with over 30 years of experience working with boards, executives and senior management in both the public and private sector health services and life sciences industries. Harold is also President of Schroeder & Schroeder Inc., a Toronto-based firm of senior program and project managers, management consultants, and corporate managers, focused on the "art and science of transformation™". Harold's clients in North America and Europe have included, among others, governments, hospitals, long-term care facilities, pharmaceutical companies, medical and assistive devices organizations, bio-technology organizations, and professional associations.

David Sibbritt is Professor of Epidemiology at the Faculty of Health, University of Technology, Sydney, Australia. David is Deputy Director of the Network of Researchers in the Public Health of Complementary and Alternative Medicine (NORPHCAM, www.norphcam.org) and is on the Executive of the "Evidence, Research and Policy in Complementary Medicine" Special Interest Group at the Public Health Association of

Australia. David is an Associate Editor for the peer-reviewed journal *BMC Health Services Research* and is on the editorial board for *Complementary Therapies in Medicine* and the *Journal of Chinese Integrative Medicine*. David has authored over 90 peer-reviewed publications and 50 conference presentations in the last 10 years. David's current research interests are predominantly in the public health of CAM, particularly related to women's health and he has an evolving interest in conducting clinical trials for CAM therapies.

Amie Steel is a PhD student at the Faculty of Health, University of Technology, Sydney, Australia, where she is also a researcher on an ARC-funded Discovery Project examining CAM use amongst pregnant women. Amie is a member of the Network of Researchers in the Public Health of Complementary and Alternative Medicine and co-founder of Embrace Holistic Services (www.embraceholistic.com). Amie is a Board Member of both the Practice Standards Committee for the Australian Register of Naturopaths and Herbalists (www.aronah.org) and the "Evidence, Research and Policy in Complementary Medicine" Special Interest Group at the Public Health Association of Australia. She is also in clinical practice as a naturopath at Herbs on the Hill (www.herbsonthehill.com.au) in Brisbane, Australia. Amie's current research focus includes a diverse area of complementary medicine including pregnancy and women's health, curriculum content of conventional and complementary medicine courses, integration and regulation of complementary medicine within the wider health system, and the interface between evidence-based medicine and complementary medicine practice.

Tobias Sundberg is a health care researcher and consultant with academic qualifications from Uppsala University, Sweden, and Karolinska Institutet, Sweden (PhD in Medical Science). In addition to his research training he has a professional background in the Swedish systems of physical therapy and massage/manual therapy, and is a European-trained osteopath. He has been an active clinician and lecturer in the fields of sports, manual, and integrative medicine since the 1990s. Tobias' main research areas and publications focus on clinical trials and comparative effectiveness research including mixed methods (quantitative and qualitative), registry studies, and health economic evaluations in conventional and integrative medicine, e.g. the investigation of conventional, manual, and complementary therapies in private practice, primary care, and hospital settings. Tobias is currently engaged as research project leader and coordinator for multiple integrative medicine studies in Sweden working for several institutions and organizations including Karolinska Institutet, IC — the Integrative Care Science Centre and Scandinavian College of Chiropractic. Tobias has been appointed with several national and international commissions of trust including assignments as temporary advisor to the World Health Organization (WHO) in Geneva, Switzerland, on the integration of traditional/complementary medicine into national health systems, lecturer in integrative medicine for decision makers and health care providers in Swedish county councils, member of the International Advisory Council for the International Journal of Therapeutic Massage and Bodywork, and scientific reviewer for journals in the fields of manual and integrative medicine including *Journal of Manipulative and Physiological Therapeutics*, *European Journal of Integrative Medicine*, and *BMC Complementary and Alternative Medicine*. In 2008 Tobias was invited by the World Federation of Chiropractic/WHO to present Swedish massage/manual therapy at the first WHO conference on manual medicine at the WHO Congress of Traditional Medicine in Beijing, China. More recently Tobias was invited to the RAND Corporation as a panelist on health economic evaluations in integrative medicine in 2011 and as a team member coordinating a health economic workshop for the International Congress for Complementary Medicine Research in London, UK, 2013.

Marissa Taylor studied at McMaster University in Hamilton, Ontario, Canada, where she received her Masters of Arts in Global Health, and a Bachelor of Arts (honours) degree in Health Studies. Marissa Taylor is currently a Program Design and Development Manager at World Vision Canada, where her specific focus and interest is on building public-private sector partnerships in Primary Health Care in a developing world context. Marissa's varied research interests include complementary and integrative medicine in cancer prevention and treatment, the examination of the social determinants of health in fragile country contexts as it relates to primary health care access and quality, and e-health technology and methods for health system strengthening in resource-poor settings. Marissa's commitment to examining the determinants of health and barriers to access and working towards creating sustainable projects that target these factors is longstanding.

Maria Costanza Torri is Assistant Professor in the Department of Sociology at the University of New Brunswick, Canada, and a member of the University's International Studies Program. She is a sociologist with strong expertise in community development and traditional medicine and has worked extensively in various countries in Latin America on environmental conservation. Following her studies in Economics at Ancona University, Italy, Maria completed two years of research at IAMM-CIHEAM in Montpellier, France. Subsequently, she completed a DEA (Diploma of Specialised Studies) and a PhD in Sociology at Paris1-Pantheon-Sorbonne, France. She was Associate Research Fellow with the Human Rights Research Centre at the University of Ottawa, Canada. Maria carried out postdoctoral research at the University of Montreal, Canada, and she has taught for the University of Toronto and Laurentian University, Canada. She has also worked extensively in 15 countries in Asia and Latin America, carrying out research projects concerning local development and traditional medicine.

Jon Wardle practices as a naturopath and he is a Chancellor's Postdoctoral Research Fellow at the University of Technology, Sydney, Australia, focusing upon workforce, regulation, and policy issues relating to CAM. Jon was previously an NHMRC Public Health PhD Scholar at the School of Population Health, University of Queensland, Australia, and a Trans-Pacific Fellow at the School of Medicine, University of Washington, USA. Jon is a founding Director of the Network of Researchers in the Public Health of Complementary and Alternative Medicine (NORPHCAM, www.norphcam.org) and is on the editorial board of several journals, including serving as the Editor-in-Chief of the *International Journal of Naturopathic Medicine* and as Associate Editor for the *Foundations of Naturopathic Medicine Project*. Jon is Co-Editor of the first evidence-based naturopathic clinical text,

Clinical Naturopathy: An Evidence-Based Guide to Practice (Churchill Livingstone, 2010) which is used as a set naturopathic text in five countries and was recently translated into Spanish. Jon lectures internationally on CAM and has several popular Australian health columns, in addition to his academic publishing endeavours.

Marjorie Weiss is the Professor of Pharmacy Practice and Medicine Use in the Department of Pharmacy and Pharmacology at the University of Bath, UK. Her research interests include how people communicate about medicines from both patient and prescriber perspective, influences on general practitioners' prescribing, patient beliefs about medicines, and the prescriber-patient interaction. With nurses and pharmacists now able to prescribe in the UK, recent work has explored how different types of health care professionals elicit patients' ideas, concerns, and expectations, and the process of sharing decisions about medicine-taking in consultation interactions. Marjorie was Principal Investigator on a recently completed Leverhulme Trust project comparing the consultations of general practitioners, nurse prescribers, and pharmacist prescribers in primary care. Having originally trained as a pharmacist, Marjorie received her DPhil from the University of Oxford, UK, and has an MSc in Social Research Methods from the University of Surrey, UK. She has a particular interest in qualitative methodologies and the use of case study research.

Kevin D. Willison obtained his PhD in Community Health from the Department of Public Health Sciences, University of Toronto, Canada. Kevin is a Lecturer at Lakehead University (Orillia campus), Canada, with the Department of Interdisciplinary Studies. He also teaches part-time with the Michener Institute for Applied Health Sciences, Toronto, Canada, and is a current Board Member of the Ontario Healthy Communities Coalition. With an interdisciplinary focus in health sociology and health services research, Kevin has presented at numerous conferences across Canada and is published in international peer-reviewed journals.

Lesley Wye is a Research Fellow at the Centre for Academic Primary Care at the University of Bristol, UK, where she carried out her PhD after employment at the King's Fund and the Department of Health, UK. She also practised as a kinesiologist for six years. Her PhD thesis explored the role of research evidence and service delivery in the mainstreaming of complementary therapies into primary care in England. She has led on other studies into complementary therapies including a feasibility study of economic evaluation of the Bristol Homeopathic Hospital and the use of homeopathic products and antibiotics in pre-school children. In addition, she has collaborated on studies on self-care in acupuncture consultations, the delivery of Alexander Technique in a hospital pain clinic, and the use of over the counter complementary therapy products. She has published findings from her complementary therapy research in journals including *Complementary Therapies in Medicine, Journal of Complementary and Alternative Medicine, Complementary Therapies in Clinical Practice, BMC Family Practice,* and *BMC Complementary and Alternative Medicine.* In addition to her interest in complementary therapies, she also leads on studies into commissioning, private healthcare, end-of-life care, and quality in community services.

Acknowledgements

The editors and publishers wish to thank the following for permission to use copyright material: BioMed Central Ltd for permission to reprint extracts from Sundberg, T., Halpin, J., Warenmark, A., and Falkenberg, T. (2007). Towards a model for integrative medicine in Swedish primary care, *BMC Health Services Research,* **7**, 107 and Sundberg, T., Petzold, M., Wandell, P., Ryden, A., and Falkenberg, T. (2009). Exploring integrative medicine for back and neck pain: A pragmatic randomized clinical pilot trial, *BMC Complementary and Alternative Medicine,* **9**, 33; Routledge for permission to reprint extracts from Broom, A. and Adams, J. (2009). "The status of complementary and alternative medicine (CAM) in biomedical education: Towards a critical engagement", in Brosnan, C. and Turner, B.S. (eds.), *Handbook of the Sociology of Medical Education*, Routledge, London, pp. 122–138; and Elsevier Ltd for permission to reprint extracts from Adams, J., Hollenberg, D., Broom, A., and Lui, C. (2009). Contextualising integration: A critical social science approach to integrative healthcare, *Journal of Manipulative and Physiological Therapeutics*, **32(9)**, 792–798.

Introduction

Patient interest in and use of complementary and alternative medicine (CAM) — a range of practices and products not traditionally associated with the medical profession or the medical curriculum including but not restricted to acupuncture, chiropractic, naturopathy, massage, and herbal medicines (Adams, 2007) — has increased exponentially over recent decades and there has been an accompanying growth in clinical, research, and policy focus upon this important area of health care (Adams *et al.*, 2012). CAM has long made its presence felt in relation to a range of conditions (often chronic and/or difficult to manage via high technology) that are the stock-in-trade of general practice and primary health care (PHC) and it comes as no surprise that the evolving relationship between CAM and the medical profession has been in large part established in the PHC setting (Adams and Tovey, 2000). Indeed, PHC — often defined as incorporating a promotional, preventive, and rehabilitative approach to a first line of patient care as provided by a multi-disciplinary team of health-care professionals working collaboratively — is potentially *able* to accommodate CAM in both conceptual and practical terms. What remains less sure is that there will be demand, acceptance, and tolerance for such an alignment of the conventional/alternative practice fields from within the ranks of conventional PHC providers, managers, and policymakers. In turn, CAM practitioners may also be less than supportive of closer ties to PHC if the requirements of developing models restrict or exclude their participation in such patient care. CAM may be perceived as holding much promise for advancing PHC, although we need to remain mindful that this is in itself a political statement that requires definitions and understandings of the ingredients and core essentials of good, effective PHC as well as CAM that are not beyond dispute (Adams and Tovey, 2000).

Integrative medicine (IM) (also known as integrative health care — perhaps a more accurate title in that it reflects what was initially a patient-led movement) and integrative models of care have been trialed and implemented in many PHC settings over the last two decades or more. Early work in the UK introduced a series of related models of integration whereby CAM services, practitioners, and/or techniques were offered alongside the work and services of those in PHC settings (Pietroni, 1992; Peters *et al.*, 1994). Meanwhile, in North America, the rise of "integrative medicine" has been closely linked to the establishment and advancement of the Consortium of Academic Health Centers for Integrative Medicine — a series of IM programs and initiatives across Canada and the US that have often evolved within departments of family medicine (amongst other fields).

It is important to acknowledge that not all integration or integrative models in PHC are the same. While some models include active participation and collaboration between CAM therapists and conventional PHC practitioners (multi-disciplinary care teams), others restrict integration to the sole responsibility and control of conventional health providers (direct or direct group integration). As these latter examples highlight, key elements to consider in IM are the political relations between professional groups and their respective control over clinical and associated decision-making.

As a core component of PHC, general practice is itself a broad church and it is not surprising that CAM and IM have been tolerated, accommodated, and even promoted from amongst the ranks of general practitioners. While the specific development and exact details of the future relationship between complementary and integrative medicine (CIM) and PHC remain unpredictable (and subject to many internal and external factors and influences), it does, nevertheless, appear reasonable to suggest that the increasing demand for CAM amongst an overwhelming number of patients (in PHC as elsewhere) is likely to lead to a "warming" and increasingly "accommodating" stance by many practitioners within PHC including general practitioners, community pharmacists, and allied health practitioners.

The research effort around this broad topic is in some ways, by wider CAM research standards, well developed. We have an emerging body of survey data, clinical research, and qualitative study exploring CAM in relation to general practice and other areas of PHC. Yet, there is much more left to explore, understand, and achieve. In broader medical and health research terms, CAM and IM in relation to PHC remains in its infancy and this collection is offered as one step, amongst many, to help address this situation. A major challenge facing those interested in investigating the territory of complementary and integrative medicine (CIM) and PHC and their intersection is research capacity building — while some in PHC research have shown research interest in the subject, this is often one interest amongst many and from a clinical perspective CIM can be viewed as simply one of a large number of competing issues facing contemporary PHC. As such, a productive and sustainable approach to researching the CIM/PHC interface requires multi-disciplinary collaborations across the CAM and conventional PHC clinical areas and broad research base.

The Book Collection

It is an interesting and important time to be examining the relationship between CIM and PHC and, while a range of pertinent issues are beginning to attract research attention, there is still much rigorous, empirical investigation required. This collection has been written and edited with this context in mind and, while a number of chapters report empirical data, other chapters are opinion pieces outlining significant practice and research issues and/or calls for the development of a research agenda to provide a further broad evidence base for the intersection of CIM/PHC practice and policy.

The book is structured into three parts. Part One introduces chapters that examine CIM use within the context of primary health care with a specific focus upon a number of practice and clinical areas. While these chapters are interested predominantly in the use and users of CIM, exploring the consumption side of the patient-practitioner perspective, they also in part (inevitably) touch upon practitioner territory examining CIM consumers' relationships and communication with providers. Extending this theme, Part Two of the collection contains chapters focused squarely upon the professional and practitioner interface between PHC and CIM. Finally, Part Three moves attention to core integrative medicine and integrative health care territory examining a grass-roots practitioner perspective of integration from within general practice, reflecting upon the dynamics and practical application of an integrative model and also critically appraising integration with regards to clinical practice and education/medical curriculum via the employment of a social science perspective. Throughout the whole book, the emphasis is upon outlining empirical findings and debate of interest across practice and research fields making it easily accessible to a multi-disciplinary audience.

While CAM consumption is certainly no longer confined to specific sub-sections of the general population in high-income countries (and CAM/traditional medicine is often the only affordable or accessible form of care available to the vast majority of the population in low-income countries), there are nevertheless a number of practice areas where CIM has attracted particularly significant patient and practitioner interest. One such area is in women's health (Adams, 2007) and, in Chapter 1, Steel and colleagues explore findings from a recent study on this topic in Australia. Drawing upon analyses from a large sample of women who report experiencing menopausal symptoms (n=853) the authors identify and discuss a number of interesting findings regarding CAM use by menopausal women within the context of PHC.

Another obvious health care area where practitioners and researchers have identified potential for CAM is with regards to chronic disease and chronic disease management. Willison and colleagues (Chapter 2) explore the potential of CAM and CAM practitioners on this topic considering approaches that could be incorporated within PHC settings to initiate or enhance chronic disease management efforts. The authors argue that CAM-related developments have the potential to help promote improvements in patient-care within PHC settings and may be feasibly deployed using an integrative medicine approach. For additional focus upon chronic disease, CIM, and PHC (general practice) also see Chapter 8 in this collection.

Concluding Part One of the book, Magin and Adams explore the relationship between general practice, CAM, and skin disease, providing an overview of CAM therapies as employed by patients with skin conditions and the prevalence of CAM use for skin disease in different clinical and non-clinical contexts (including general practice). Drawing upon the example of atopic eczema the authors explore the centrality of CAM-GP relationships especially with regards to evidence of efficacy, adverse effects, quality control, and ethics around this topic.

Chapter 4 explores the current and potential role of naturopaths for providing PHC services in areas of unmet need. Drawing primarily upon the situation in the Australian health care system, Wardle and Adams argue that while the incorporation of naturopaths into PHC may bring benefits, it also presents challenges associated with practitioner variability and patient risk. Nevertheless, with the development of appropriate regulatory and quality policies, this health care resource may attract careful attention amongst other options with regards to future PHC policy and service planning in countries in which naturopaths have a major presence.

Examining the use of traditional medicine in low-income countries, Hollenberg and Torri (Chapter 5) investigate the role of local health traditions (in this case home herbal gardens in India) in promoting health security. The authors contest that traditional medicine must be considered a legitimate and coherent system of locally embedded healing knowledge with relevance to the local communities if it is to be most effectively used and its potential harnessed.

Meanwhile, in Chapter 6, Wardle and colleagues consider the relationship and interface between general practice and CIM in rural health care and provision. An in-depth understanding of CIM use and practice in rural health, the authors argue, helps to provide insights for a number of rural health care issues which have not received substantial attention to date. These include care-seeking patterns, the realities of healthcare delivery, networks and provision management, as well as barriers to services in these locations. Furthermore, the prevalence of CIM use in rural communities highlights the potential volume and scope of health seeking behaviour and activity in rural settings which have significant implications for health service management and planning but have to date escaped empirical investigation. Further understanding of such CAM use and practice is essential in aiding the informed decision-making of rural practitioners, patients and policymakers with regards to both CAM and wider conventional care options.

A major component of contemporary CAM is over-the-counter products. Herbal medicines, dietary supplements and vitamins are increasingly available from a wide range of sources (health food stores, community pharmacies, supermarkets) and one interesting dynamic of this development is the extent to which patients seek advice and professional guidance for such consumption (both in terms of CAM and conventional PHC professionals). In Chapter 7, Cramer and colleagues report findings from an ethnographic study of the sale and purchase of CAM over-the-counter products in community pharmacies and health shops from the perspective of relative expertise. As the authors point out, community pharmacies and health shops are examples of first-contact PHC and the chapter aims to address a crucial question: when it comes to buying over-the-counter CAM products just *who* is the expert: customers or shop staff or medical practitioners?

Part Three of the collection turns more squarely upon the integration of alternatives within core PHC territory and practice. For example, Peters (Chapter 8) explores the possible role of CAM adoption and integration within general practice as a means of addressing three important challenges facing PHC: cost, care, and commitment. Promoting an insider perspective, he also argues the exploration of self-care and CAM may support doctors' engagement with the essential "art of medicine" — an element viewed by many to be missing from contemporary general practice and PHC more broadly.

Despite the many IM models and initiatives underway there remain a number of core challenges facing those who lead the charge towards an integrative model of PHC. In Chapter 9, Sundberg provides a brief overview and research summary of a Swedish PHC project developing, implementing, and evaluating a model for IM with specific focus upon the management of low back pain and neck pain. Undertaking an explorative mixed method study, Sundberg explores the relevance of IM as a health service option in Swedish PHC concluding that the study findings attest to the need to further investigate IM as a complex healthcare intervention and to continue to explore relevant combinations of outcomes to help understand the relevance of IM in primary health care.

Chapter 10, closing the collection, moves a further step in critically appraising IM, in this case in terms of both practice and medical education. Adams and colleagues subject IM and IM models to a critical social science perspective in order to consider what is actually occurring interprofessionally between biomedicine (general practice/PHC) and CAM within grassroots as well as wider socio-historical contexts, and to move beyond simplistic notions and models of integration that suggest a coming together of practices and/or practitioners and a sense that there is more linearity to health care delivery across the modalities available. As Adams and colleagues suggest, the employment of a critical social science perspective and situating the development of IM in wider socio-political parameters and in processes of struggles for professionalization and legitimacy enable us to view the evolution of integrative health care and education, and the relationship between conventional and alternative medicine, as far from smooth and linear — a perspective that helps provide a broader picture of the power and politics involved in the IM movement.

References

Adams, J. (ed.) (2007). *Researching Complementary and Alternative Medicine*, Routledge, London.

Adams, J., Andrews, G., Barnes, J., Broom, A., and Magin, P. (eds.) (2012). *Traditional, Complementary and Integrative Medicine: An International Reader*, Palgrave, Basingstoke.

Adams, J. and Tovey, P. (2000). "Complementary medicine and primary care: Towards a grassroots focus", in Tovey, P. (ed.), *Contemporary Primary Care: The Challenges of Change*, Open University Press, Buckingham.

Peters, D., Davies, P., and Pietroni, P. (1994). Musculo-skeletal clinic in general practice: A study of one years' referrals, *British Journal of General Practice,* **44**, 25–29.

Pietroni, P. (1992). Beyond the boundaries: Relationship between general practice and complementary medicine, *British Medical Journal,* **305**, 564–566.

Part One

**Patients, Illness and Disease:
CIM Use and its Context in Primary
Health Care**

CHAPTER 1

Primary Health Care, Complementary and Alternative Medicine and Women's Health: A Focus upon Menopause

Amie Steel, Jane Frawley, Jon Adams,
David Sibbritt, and Alex Broom

1.1 Introduction

Australian women are integrating primary health care (PHC) and complementary and alternative medicine (CAM) to alleviate a range of symptoms and conditions. This chapter introduces the use of CAM for women's health in general and more particularly, explores the integration of CAM alongside mainstream PHC by women during the menopause (Xue *et al.*, 2007; Adams *et al.*, 2003).

It has been argued that the trend identifying women as higher users of CAM is unsurprising as women also use conventional health care services more frequently than men (Beal, 1998). Research examining the general Australian population suggests that some women use acupuncture (9.6%), chiropractic (17.1%) and osteopathy (5.8%) as part of their health management. However, research has only provided preliminary investigation of the specific usage patterns of Australian women. One study (Adams *et al.*, 2007) estimates that 11% of mid-age Australian women consult with naturopaths and herbalists and that these women are more likely to live in non-urban areas, and in contrast with the general population, are less likely to have completed post-secondary education. Adams *et al.* (2007) also identified these women using naturopaths and herbalists as likely to experience symptoms of both general health complaints (back pain (53%), stiff or painful joints (50%), allergies (45%) and severe tiredness (43%), as well as symptoms related to women's health (hot flushes (50%) and night sweats (37%)). Consistent with the general population these women appear to be engaging with both conventional PHC and CAM practitioners (Rayner *et al.*, 2009; Stankiewicz *et al.*, 2007). The reasons for women's integration of CAM and PHC are complex but some trends have been observed. For example, a lack of satisfaction with biomedical care tends to be associated with higher CAM use for women (Adams *et al.*, 2011a), except in rural communities with some research suggesting CAM use is linked to poorer access to conventional PHC (Adams *et al.*, 2011b) rather than dissatisfaction with conventional care. When viewed in conjunction with the high CAM use amongst women, this reinforces the potential PHC role of CAM practitioners and treatments. It also suggests that, given the high number of female CAM users with menopause-related symptoms such as hot flushes and night sweats, an examination of the relationship between PHC utilisation and CAM use amongst menopausal women is warranted.

1.1.1 *The rise of CAM use in menopause*

Emerging international data identifies high levels of CAM use by women for the management of menopausal symptoms. Recent data suggests 80% of menopausal women (n = 3,302) in the US have used some form of CAM in the previous six years for symptom control (Bair *et al.*, 2008), and another US study (n = 1,206) found that almost 50% of women used alternative treatments for symptom management, the most popular being diet/nutrition, exercise/yoga, relaxation/stress management and homeopathic/naturopathic remedies (Daley *et al.*, 2006). Rates of CAM use elsewhere in the world have also been found to be high with 91% of women in Canada and 82.5% in Australia using CAM during the period of menopausal transition (Lunny and Fraser, 2010; Gollschewski *et al.*, 2004). Another Australian study found that 53.8% of women had used a CAM product and/or consulted a CAM practitioner for the relief of menopausal symptoms during the previous 12 months (van der Sluijs *et al.*, 2007). Other studies have found that 33.5% of Italian women utilise CAM during menopause along with 43% of menopausal women in the UK who employed over-the-counter nutritional supplements (Cardini *et al.*, 2010; Gokhale *et al.*, 2003).

Differences in prevalence rates of CAM across cultures and studies may be due, at least in part, to varying definitions of CAM and time frames employed. However, regardless of these differences, current CAM usage during menopausal transition appears significant. Bair *et al.* (2008) examined the use of CAM during menopause transition and whether there were any variations in utilisation due to ethnicity (Bair *et al.*, 2008). The authors reported that around 80% of all participants had used some form of CAM during the six-year study period. White and Japanese women had the highest prevalence of use (60%), followed by Chinese (46%), African American (40%) and Hispanic (20%) women. White women were not found to alter their use of CAM as they transitioned through menopause, whilst Chinese and African American women increased their CAM use as they transitioned to perimenopause and decreased usage in postmeno-pause. Hispanic and Japanese women were found to decrease use in early perimenopause, increase use as they transitioned into late perimenopause and decrease use again as they proceeded to postmenopause.

Common drivers of general CAM use such as previous CAM use, tertiary education, age, health beliefs, symptom sensitivity, personal experience and health co-morbidities (Bair *et al.*, 2002; 2005; 2008; Gold *et al.*, 2007; Gollschewski *et al.*, 2005; Lunny and Fraser, 2010) are also pertinent during menopause. A US study found that women who commonly used CAM for menopausal symptoms were higher conventional health care users when compared with non-users of CAM (Bair *et al.*, 2005). Another study identified women who use herbal medicines as more likely to: experience good overall health, be under 55 years of age, have previously (but not currently) used hormone replacement therapy (HRT) and to have carried out breast self-examinations in the last two years (Gollschewski *et al.*, 2005).

1.1.2 *CAM products and practices commonly used in menopause*

Complementary medicines such as soy products and herbal medicines are commonly used during the menopause to control problematic symptoms.

Randomised clinical trials (RCTs) of soy products have found both positive (Scambia *et al.*, 2000; Upmalis *et al.*, 2000; Faure *et al.*, 2002; Albert *et al.*, 2002; Crisafulli *et al.*, 2004; Nahas *et al.*, 2007) and negative findings (MacGregor *et al.*, 2005; Burke *et al.*, 2003; Nikander *et al.*, 2005; Knight *et al.*, 2001). These conflicting results may be due to large variations that exist in the isoflavone content of soy products (Boniglia *et al.*, 2009).

A recent review examined the evidence from systematic reviews, RCTs and epidemiological studies and found that while phytoestrogen-containing products may have only minimal benefits for hot flushes, they may nevertheless provide other positive health effects such as reducing plasma lipid levels and bone loss (Borrelli and Ernst, 2010). Black cohosh (*Cimicifuga racemosa/Actaea racemosa*), red clover (*Trifolium pratense*) and hops (*Humulus lupulus*) are amongst the most common herbal remedies utilised during menopause. It is believed that these herbs exhibit hormonal modulating effects through various mechanisms. Black cohosh has attracted the most rigorous investigation for the treatment of hot flushes in menopause and overall, RCTs have been positive (Borrelli and Ernst, 2010; Cheema *et al.*, 2007). However, many difficulties exist in herbal medicine research alongside, and in addition to, the normal methodological considerations of a rigorous RCT, such as quality of the herb material, dose, standardisation and phytoequivalence issues.

1.1.3 *A time for integration?*

The symptoms of menopause are primarily managed by a general practitioner (GP), as opposed to a specialist. Previous research has shown quite clearly that women would like to gain information on all facets of menopause including CAM use from their GP in order to make informed choices (Armitage *et al.*, 2007), and are often dissatisfied with the information they are given (Sayakhot *et al.*, 2011). Women report several frustrating challenges when gathering information about the menopause, namely a lack of time to gather this information, a dearth of relevant information and poor information quality. These challenges may be exacerbated by limited consultation times with their GPs to discuss information related to their condition in sufficient detail (Taylor, 2009).

Additionally, these women also express an interest in material relating to the general menopausal process and conventional and CAM treatments, including information on safety.

Health care professionals such as GPs are ideally placed to advise women about the safe use of CAM during the menopause. However, many have often had very limited training in complementary medicine and may not feel confident recommending or prescribing such treatments (Pirotta *et al.*, 2011), and despite some evidence that CAM practitioners are attempting to provide a bridge between conventional medicine and CAM practice (Wardle, 2010), this is still the exception rather than the rule.

Unfortunately, menopausal women do not appear to be disclosing their use of CAM to their conventional care providers (Wade *et al.*, 2008), which may be due to patients' perceptions that doctors hold a negative attitude towards CAM and are likely to be judgemental or disinterested (Robinson and McGrail, 2004). Pharmacists are also in a prime position to offer advice on the use of complementary medicines for the menopause. Most pharmacies supply both conventional and complementary medications, enabling the pharmacist to advise on the use of CAM products and check any potential interactions with prescription medication, a service preferred by pharmacy customers (Braun *et al.*, 2010) and considered important by pharmacists (National Prescribing Service, 2010) (also see Chapter 7 for a more detailed discussion of the role of pharmacists in CAM consumption). This chapter will now focus upon the findings from a recent study examining the integration of PHC providers and CAM for the management of symptoms during the menopausal transition.

1.2 Methods

1.2.1 *Sample*

The survey data analysed in this chapter is from a substudy of the Australian Longitudinal Survey on Women's Health (ALSWH). The ALSWH was designed to investigate multiple factors affecting the health and well-being of a cohort of women over a 20-year period. Women in three age groups ("young" 18–23, "mid-age" 45–50 and "older" 70–75 years) were randomly selected from the national Medicare database (Brown *et al.*, 1998).

The baseline survey, Survey 1 (n = 14,779), was conducted in 1996 and the respondents have been shown to be broadly representative of the national population of women in the target age groups (Brown *et al.*, 1999). The focus of this substudy is women from the mid-age cohort. A total of 2,120 women who had indicated in Survey 5 (2007) that they consulted a CAM practitioner were sent a questionnaire, of which 1,800 women completed and returned. From these 1,800 respondents, 853 women indicated that they had consulted a CAM practitioner in the previous 12 months (July 2008–July 2009) and that they were experiencing menopausal symptoms. It is these women that were included in the analyses for this study. Relevant ethical approval was gained from the Human Ethics Committee at the University of Queensland and University of Newcastle, Australia.

1.2.2 *Demographic characteristics*

The address of usual residence at each survey for each woman in the ALSWH has been geo-coded and allocated an ARIA+ remoteness score according to the ASGC (Australian Standard Geographical Classification) Remoteness Areas classification released in 2001 by the Australian Bureau of Statistics (Australian Institute of Health and Welfare, 2004). The ASGC classification categorises areas of residence as "major cities", "inner regional", "outer regional", "remote" and "very remote", based on road distance from a locality to the closest service centre. The participants of this study were categorised into four areas of residence: major cities (ARIA+ score: 0–0.20), inner regional (>0.20–2.40), outer regional (>2.40–5.92) and remote/very remote (>5.92). The women were asked about their current marital status. A measure of the women's disposable income was obtained from a question asking how they managed on the income available to them.

1.2.3 *Rating of health care providers/services*

The women were asked to rate their level of satisfaction with various aspects of conventional health care providers (such as access to a female GP, hours when a GP is available, outcomes of medical care, quality of care provided). Each aspect was rated via a five-point Likert scale, where 1 = excellent and 5 = poor. The women were also asked their level of agreement to a series of statements regarding alternative medicine (such as "An alternative health practitioner spends a longer time with me in consultation compared with my doctor", "I find it easier to talk to an alternative health practitioner than to a doctor"). Each statement was rated via a five-point Likert scale, where 1 = strongly agree and 5 = strongly disagree.

1.2.4 *Information sources for alternative medicine*

The women were provided with a list of information sources and asked to indicate if any were influential in their decision to use alternative medicine. The list included: family or relative, partner, friend or colleague, Internet, book or magazine, mass media, doctor, pharmacist, allied health worker and alternative health practitioner.

1.2.5 *Communication*

The women were asked if they informed their doctor or a pharmacist before or after using alternative medicine.

1.2.6 *Use of CAM*

The women were asked if they had consulted with a range of CAM practitioners in the previous 12 months. The list of CAM practitioners included: massage therapist, chiropractor, herbalist/naturopath, meditation/yoga therapist, acupuncturist, osteopath, reflexologist, spiritual health therapist, homeopath, traditional Chinese medicine therapist, aromatherapist, Ayurveda practitioner and music therapist. The women were also asked if they had used a range of self-prescribed alternative treatments. This list of alternative treatments included: herbal medicines, vitamins or minerals, meditation or yoga, aromatherapy oils, Chinese medicine and prayer or spiritual healing.

1.2.7 *Statistical analyses*

Frequencies and percentages were used to describe the responses to questionnaire items. All analyses were conducted using the statistical software SAS 9.1 (SAS, 2006).

1.3 Results

The women's consultation patterns with alternative health practitioners in the previous 12 months are presented in Table 1.1.

It can be seen that massage therapists were clearly the most popular practitioner group consulted, with 76% of women consulting a massage therapist at least once in the previous 12 months, including 21% consulting a massage therapist seven or more times. Similarly, chiropractors were consulted by 54% of women within the previous 12 months and mostly (21%) seven or more times during that period. Herbalist/naturopaths were also highly consulted, with 34% of women consulting a herbalist/naturopath at least once in the previous 12 months, but commonly (18%) only once or twice in that period. Other popular practitioner groups consulted were meditation/yoga practitioners and acupuncturists, 24% and 20% respectively in the previous 12 months.

Table 1.1 Consultations with alternative health practitioners in the previous 12 months.

	Number of consultations in previous 12 months				
	None	1 or 2	3 or 4	5 or 6	7 or more
Alternative health practitioner	%	%	%	%	%
Acupuncturist	80	10	3	2	5
Aromatherapist	94	4	1	0	1
Ayurveda practitioner	98	1	1	0	0
Chiropractor	46	14	11	8	21
Herbalist/Naturopath	66	18	7	5	4
Homeopath	89	6	2	1	2
Massage therapist	24	28	16	11	21
Meditation/Yoga	76	3	4	2	15
Music therapist	98	1	0	0	1
Osteopath	86	5	3	2	4
Reflexologist	86	8	2	1	3
Spiritual health therapist	86	7	2	1	4
Traditional Chinese medicine therapist	90	6	1	1	2
Other	85	3	4	3	5

Table 1.2 Self-prescribed treatments used in the previous 12 months.

	Number of times used in previous 12 months				
	None	1 or 2	3 or 4	5 or 6	7 or more
Self-prescribed treatment	%	%	%	%	%
Herbal medicines	44	12	7	4	33
Vitamins/minerals	10	8	7	3	72
Meditation or yoga	68	3	2	4	23
Aromatherapy oils	64	11	7	4	14
Chinese medicine	89	4	2	1	4
Prayer or spiritual healing	64	5	4	2	25
Other alternative treatments	88	1	1	1	9

Table 1.2 shows the women's use of self-prescribed alternative treatments in the previous 12 months. Vitamins/minerals were consumed by 90% of women, with the majority (72%) consuming vitamins/minerals seven or more times in the 12-month period. Herbal medicines were another popular self-prescribed treatment, with 56% of women consuming them at least once in the previous 12 months, including 33% of women who consumed these medicines seven or more times in the 12-month period. Meditation or yoga and prayer or spiritual healing were other common, regularly used self-prescribed CAM treatments, with 23% and 25% of women using these treatments seven or more times in a one-year period, respectively.

In terms of communicating the use of alternative medicine with their primary health providers, only 11% of women would always (32% sometimes, 25% rarely, 32% never) inform their doctor *before* using alternative medicines, while 24% of women would always (43% sometimes, 17% rarely, 16% never) inform their doctor *after* using alternative medicines. Similarly, only 10% of women would always (27% sometimes, 22% rarely, 41% never) inform their pharmacist *before* using alternative medicines, while 8% of women would always (19% sometimes, 19% rarely, 54% never) inform their pharmacist *after* using alternative medicines.

The information sources that were influential in the women's decision to use alternative medicines were numerous. The most common influential information sources were friend or colleague (41%), family or relative (39%)

and book or magazine (28%). Primary health providers were less influential, with 27% of women stating influence from their doctor, 14% from their pharmacist and 4% from an allied health worker. Alternative health practitioners were influential for 26% of women; the Internet and mass media were only influential for 7% and 12% of women respectively.

The women's attitudes towards alternative medicine and doctors are presented in Table 1.3. Overwhelmingly, 90% of women agreed or

Table 1.3 Attitudes towards alternative medicine and doctors.

Statement	Strongly agree %	Agree %	Neutral %	Disagree %	Strongly disagree %
An alternative health practitioner spends a longer time with me in consultation, compared with my doctor	17	29	39	14	1
An alternative health practitioner provides more support to me than my doctor does	12	17	46	22	3
I find it easier to talk to an alternative health practitioner than to a doctor	10	19	42	25	4
I have a more equal relationship with alternative health practitioners than with doctors	9	19	44	25	3
I have difficulty accessing conventional medicine	2	8	24	50	16
Doctors should be able to advise their patients about commonly used alternative medicines	25	65	8	2	0

strongly agreed that doctors should be able to provide them with advice about commonly used alternative medicines. Nearly half (46%) of the women agreed or strongly agreed that alternative health practitioners spend more time with them in consultation, compared with their doctor. A similar percentage of women agreed or disagreed to the statements: their alternative health practitioner provides more support than their doctor, they find it easier to talk to an alternative health practitioner than a doctor and they have a more equal relationship with alternative health practitioners than with doctors. The majority of women disagreed (50%) or strongly disagreed (16%) with the statement that they have difficulty accessing conventional medicine.

Table 1.4 presents the women's rating of access to and satisfaction with their GP. Positive assessment was provided by the majority of women in

Table 1.4 Access to and satisfaction with general practitioners.

Statement	Excellent %	Very good %	Good %	Fair %	Poor %
Access to a female GP	19	23	28	17	13
Hours when a GP is available	7	22	35	27	9
Number of GPs you have to choose from	10	25	32	20	13
Ease of seeing the GP of your choice	9	22	28	26	15
How long you wait to get a GP appointment	7	19	30	27	17
Quality of care provided by your GP	24	37	31	8	0
Amount of time for a GP consultation	14	28	34	20	4
Amount of information sharing by GP	17	31	33	16	3
The outcomes of your medical care (how much you are helped)	15	33	36	14	2
The personal manner of your GP	34	36	24	5	1
The technical skills of your GP	30	37	25	7	1

relation to matters of access, where: 70% of women rated their access to a female GP as being excellent, very good or good; 67% rated the number of GPs they have to choose from as excellent, very good or good; 64% rated the hours when a GP is available as excellent, very good or good; 59% rated the ease of seeing a GP of choice as excellent, very good or good and 56% rated how long they had to wait to get a GP appointment as excellent, very good or good. Similarly, the satisfaction of GP care was also highly rated (excellent, very good or good) as was the personal manner of their GP (92%), the quality of care provided by their GP (92%), the technical skills of their GP (92%), the outcomes of their medical care (84%), the amount of information sharing by their GP (81%) and the amount of time for a GP consultation (76%).

1.4 Discussion

This study identifies a number of interesting findings regarding CAM use by menopausal women within the context of PHC. One such finding is the consultation patterns with CAM practitioners. In particular, the various approaches to the practice of different alternative health practitioner groups may be highlighted by the various consultation patterns identified. For example, the high frequency of consultations to massage therapists, reported in our study, may reflect a tendency for women who visit massage therapists to feel the benefit of massage is best achieved by ongoing treatment to maintain physical and mental relaxation, an approach often encouraged by proponents of massage therapy (Smith *et al.*, 2009). Likewise, the high overall rate of massage use may reflect the perception that massage is used for prevention and as a self-care strategy for general well-being as well as for specific musculoskeletal conditions (Smith *et al.*, 2009).

Similarly, women who visited chiropractors tended to do so frequently over a 12-month period. This pattern also reflects an approach to regular maintenance advocated by chiropractors through an average of 14 visits per year (Rupert, 2000). Whilst also similar, the higher frequency of attending yoga or meditation may simply reflect the structure of yoga/ meditation being offered in class formats over defined time periods (Booth-LaForce *et al.*, 2007; Javnbakht *et al.*, 2009; Manocha *et al.*, 2007). It may also signal a perception amongst the women that, similar to the case of massage and chiropractic care, the value and benefit of yoga or meditation is only achieved after recurrent practice (Hari Kaur Khalsa, 2004). Comparable findings have been identified for massage, chiropractic care and yoga/meditation in other demographic groups such as pregnant women (Adams *et al.*, 2009), women with health conditions such as cancer (Rees *et al.*, 2000), as well as women in general (Factor-Litvak *et al.*, 2001), suggesting that these views are not unique to menopausal women but rather to the particular CAM therapies.

In contrast to the massage, chiropractic and yoga professional groups who were visited frequently, the other CAM practitioners were consulted less often over the 12-month period of this study. This was particularly pronounced for acupuncturists and herbalist/naturopaths — a finding which has been reported elsewhere (Newton *et al.*, 2002). The different pattern identified here may be due to a perception amongst the women that the value in these professional groups is only for treatment rather than maintenance and as such only require sufficient consultations to remediate their presenting complaint. Alternatively, this pattern may reflect the approach of the practitioners such as herbalist/naturopaths to allow more time between consultations for women to integrate diet and lifestyle changes (Wardle, 2010).

Vitamins/minerals, herbal medicines and meditation/yoga are self-prescribed treatments which were commonly and regularly used. Vitamins and minerals have consistently been found to be popular in the international literature, with an Australian study finding that 49% of women had used nutritional supplements to control menopausal symptoms (Gollschewski *et al.*, 2004). In addition, 28.8% used a vitamin E supplement and 34% used evening primrose oil. A UK study (n = 326) also reported a high prevalence of supplement use with 44% of women using vitamins and 53% using evening primrose oil (Gokhale *et al.*, 2003), and this study found that 71% (n = 242) of women were users of conventional HRT and of these, 46% were also using food supplements such as phytoestrogens. Our study reported a very high usage of vitamins/minerals with 90% of women using these supplements within the previous 12 months and the majority (72%) consuming vitamins/minerals seven or more times in the 12-month period. It is conceivable that a reasonable proportion of these women could also be using HRT; this is quite possibly innocuous. However, research needs to be conducted to ascertain exactly what supplements women are taking and to confirm the safety of their consumption.

Influential information sources utilised by the menopausal women regarding CAM were found to be friends or colleagues, family or relatives and books or magazines. Conventional PHC providers were found to be less influential. This is a fairly common theme amongst research papers reporting on women's information sources for the use of CAM during the menopause (Gokhale *et al.*, 2003; Armitage *et al.*, 2007; Hill-Sakurai *et al.*, 2008), and whilst it is consistent for women to source information on CAM from family and friends, it is perhaps concerning that they are more influenced by information and advice acquired via these sources than from conventional health care practitioners. Armitage *et al.* (2007) found that most women who responded to their survey (n = 413) favoured evidence-based information despite a substantial number also relying on personal accounts from friends and family (Armitage *et al.*, 2007). The two different types of information sourcing were not found to be mutually exclusive as many respondents indicated that they preferred and utilised both sources of information.

The Internet and the mass media were not found to have a significant influence on women's treatment decisions on the use of CAM for menopausal symptoms. This may be related to the age of the women and the possibility that in general they may use computers and online social networking less than younger women. PHC professionals such as GPs and pharmacists are well positioned to enquire regarding women's CAM use during the menopause. Women in our study have indicated a desire for their conventional PHC practitioner to provide advice about commonly used CAM and this may indeed raise an important educational/training need for GPs.

The women in our study were found to be unlikely to communicate use of alternative medicine to their doctor prior to their use of CAM products and treatments or consultations with CAM therapists. This finding is supported by previous research which report high rates of disclosure to conventional care providers for a range of health conditions but comparatively low disclosure for women with menopausal symptoms (Wade *et al.*, 2008). This previous study did not differentiate between the timing of disclosure, and our findings suggest the women were somewhat more likely to inform the doctor of their CAM use after consumption. The possible reasons for this non-disclosure of CAM use to medical practitioners has been reported elsewhere in the literature where patients may avoid disclosure due to fear of judgement by the medical practitioner, or perceptions that the doctor would not understand or was simply not interested (Robinson and McGrail, 2004). Others have suggested that patients perceive their use of CAM to be unimportant or not relevant to the doctor (Eisenberg *et al.*, 2001). Whilst our study identified that the women perceived that doctors should be able to provide them with advice about commonly used CAM, it does not provide insights into whether they perceived their own doctor to hold sufficient knowledge or whether this contributed to limit their disclosure. Based upon the previous research on this topic (Eisenberg *et al.*, 2001; Robinson and McGrail, 2004) it is also possible that poor disclosure may be encouraged due to a failure on behalf of the doctor to enquire about CAM use.

Similar to doctors, women also reported low rates of disclosure regarding CAM use to their pharmacists. Whilst this may also reflect some of the issues identified above regarding perceived poor receptivity to the topic, it may also highlight a lower importance placed on pharmacists as members of the woman's team of health professionals, although there is an absence of previous research on this topic. This is a potential concern as pharmacists are a front-line health practitioner in the community who, alongside doctors, provide front-line PHC in the community (see Chapter 7 for a more detailed discussion). Available data does suggest pharmacy customers believe pharmacists should provide information and recommendations on CAM products or employ a qualified CAM practitioner, but previous work does not examine participants' disclosure practices with regards to CAM (Braun *et al.*, 2010). A recent survey of pharmacists conducted by the National Prescribing Service reported a substantial number (85.5%) considered it important to ask patients if they were taking CAM products (National Prescribing Service, 2010), suggesting that the attitude of the pharmacists may not be a barrier to disclosure although this does not discount the possibility that women may perceive pharmacists to hold negative attitudes towards CAM. Unfortunately, the current research does not provide any further insights into this issue. This absence of data is of particular concern when considering the high rate of self-prescription reported in this chapter, as many over-the-counter CAM products are sold in pharmacies. Given the shared location it is curious that women are not disclosing their CAM product use to their pharmacist at the time of purchasing their CAM product or prescription medicine. The absence of disclosure of CAM use by women to either their doctor or pharmacist is a missed opportunity for PHC practitioners to provide information and guidance, particularly for those women self-prescribing CAM. As such, avenues to encourage disclosure need to be examined to fully realise the potential benefit of patient-clinician interactions with regard to CAM for these two practitioner groups.

Women in our study reported satisfaction with the care provided by their GP and had no concerns with access to GP services. This trend suggests that women are receiving the care they expect from their GP and as such are accessing CAM practitioner services for reasons beyond dissatisfaction with conventional care. This is not entirely consistent with the findings of previous research focusing specifically upon women's experience of GP care related to menopause and breast cancer (Sayakhot et al., 2011). Dissatisfaction with the menopause information provided at the time of diagnosis was quite high amongst our study participants with nearly half less than satisfied with the general menopause information (46%) and potential fertility information (45%) and 74% dissatisfied with the information about long-term complications of menopause. Women may instead be seeking CAM to treat conditions which are not generally managed well by conventional care such as musculoskeletal conditions and mental health problems (Featherstone et al., 2003), or due to concerns about the safety of hormonal treatment for menopausal symptoms (Buick et al., 2005). Women may also be using CAM to promote general health and well-being (Goh et al., 2009) and to prevent (Wardle et al., 2010), rather than to treat, a current condition.

Our study also found that women perceive CAM practitioners as spending more time with them in consultation compared with their doctor. This perception may be one of the drivers supporting the high use of CAM by menopausal women. Previous research has identified that CAM users value the time allocated in consultation by CAM practitioners, the personal empowerment afforded by engagement with CAM, and the focus on individualised and unique care (Wardle et al., 2010; Bishop et al., 2010). Research has indicated that an aspect which underpins this approach is the philosophical values held by CAM users which promote wellness and self-care (Caspi *et al.*, 2004; Bishop *et al.*, 2007). Alongside this philosophy is also argued to be a broader view which asserts that individuals are entitled to, and deserving of, allocated time to nourish and nurture self, and that control of the health care process resides with the individual rather than the clinician (Bishop *et al.*, 2007). This research in the more general population is also supported by findings from menopausal women (Gollschewski *et al.*, 2007). In stark contrast to the time invested by CAM practitioners to the attention of individual patients, is the scarcity of time allowed by conventional care providers which may affect their ability to provide patient-centred care (Taylor, 2009). The disparity in experiences between CAM and conventional medicine is potentially highlighted more profoundly by the recent movement towards individuals identifying themselves more as "health consumers" rather than "patients" (Berenson and Cassel, 2009).

The interpretation of the findings reported here is potentially limited by the fact that the participants' use of CAM and GPs was self-reported. Despite this, the ALSWH is a respected source of data for epidemiological research relating to women's health in Australia, and this limitation is outweighed by the opportunities provided from conducting an analysis of the patterns of use, information sources and communication dynamics with GPs regarding CAM use by menopausal women.

Acknowledgements

The research on which this chapter was based was conducted as part of the ALSWH which is funded by the Australian Government Department of Health and Ageing (DOHA). We are grateful to the DOHA for funding and to the women who provided the survey data. We also thank the NHMRC who funded this research via grant #511181 and NHMRC Career Development Award for Professor Jon Adams.

References

Adams, J., Lui, C., Sibbritt, D., Broom, A., Wardle, J., Homer, C., and Beck, S. (2009). Women's use of complementary and alternative medicine during pregnancy: A critical review of the literature, *Birth*, **36**, 237–245.

Adams, J., Sibbritt, D., and Lui, C. (2011a). The urban-rural divide in complementary and alternative medicine use: A longitudinal study of 10,638 women, *BMC Complementary and Alternative Medicine*, **11**, 2.

Adams, J., Sibbritt, D., and Young, A.F. (2007). Consultations with a naturopath or herbalist: The prevalence of use and profile of users amongst mid-aged women in Australia, *Public Health*, **121**, 954–957.

Adams, J., Sibbritt, D., Broom, A., Loxton, D., Pirotta, M., Humphreys, J., and Lui, C. (2011b). A comparison of complementary and alternative medicine users and use across geographical areas: A national survey of 1,427 women, *BMC Complementary and Alternative Medicine*, **11**, 85.

Adams, J., Sibbritt, D., Easthope, G., and Young, A. (2003). The profile of women who consult alternative health practitioners in Australia, *Medical Journal of Australia*, **179**, 297–300.

Albert, A., Altabre, C., Baro, F., Buendia, E., Cabero, A., Cancelo, M.J., Castelo-Branco, C., Chantre, P., Duran, M., Haya, J., Imbert, P., Julia, D., Lanchares, J.L., Llaneza, P., Manubens, M., Minano, A., Quereda, F., Ribes, C., and Vazquez, F. (2002). Efficacy and safety of a phytoestrogen preparation derived from Glycine max (L.) Merr in climacteric symptomatology: A multicentric, open, prospective and non-randomized trial, *Phytomedicine*, **9**, 85–92.

Armitage, G.D., Suter, E., Verhoef, M.J., Bockmuehl, C., and Bobey, M. (2007). Women's needs for CAM information to manage menopausal symptoms, *Climacteric*, **10**, 215–224.

Australian Institute of Health and Welfare (2004). *Rural, Regional and Remote Health: A Guide to Remoteness Classification*, Canberra, Australian Institute of Health and Welfare.

Bair, Y.A., Gold, E.B., Azari, R.A., Greendale, G., Sternfeld, B., Harkey, M.R., and Kravitz, R.L. (2005). Use of conventional and complementary health care during the transition to menopause: Longitudinal results from the Study of Women's Health Across the Nation (SWAN), *Menopause*, **12**, 31–39.

Bair, Y.A., Gold, E.B., Greendale, G.A., Sternfeld, B., Adler, S.R., Azari, R., and Harkey, M. (2002). Ethnic differences in use of complementary and alternative medicine at midlife: Longitudinal results from SWAN participants, *American Journal of Public Health*, **92**, 1832–1840.

Bair, Y.A., Gold, E.B., Zhang, G., Rasor, N., Utts, J., Upchurch, D.M., Chyu, L., Greendale, G.A., Sternfeld, B., and Adler, S.R. (2008). Use of complementary and alternative medicine during the menopause transition: Longitudinal results from the Study of Women's Health Across the Nation, *Menopause*, **15**, 32–43.

Beal, M.W. (1998). Women's use of complementary and alternative therapies in reproductive health care, *Journal of Nurse Midwifery*, **43**, 224–234.

Berenson, R.A. and Cassel, C.K. (2009). Consumer-driven health care may not be what patients need-caveat emptor, *Journal of the American Medical Association*, **301**, 321–323.

Bishop, F.L., Yardley, L., and Lewith, G.T. (2007). A systematic review of beliefs involved in the use of complementary and alternative medicine, *Journal of Health Psychology*, **12**, 851.

Bishop, F.L., Yardley, L., and Lewith, G.T. (2010). Why consumers maintain complementary and alternative medicine use: A qualitative study, *The Journal of Alternative and Complementary Medicine*, **16**, 175–182.

Boniglia, C., Carratù, B., Gargiulo, R., Giammarioli, S., Mosca, M., and Sanzini, E. (2009). Content of phytoestrogens in soy-based dietary supplements, *Food Chemistry*, **115**, 1389–1392.

Booth-LaForce, C., Thurston, R.C., and Taylor, M.R. (2007). A pilot study of a hatha yoga treatment for menopausal symptoms, *Maturitas*, **57**, 286–295.

Borrelli, F. and Ernst, E. (2010). Alternative and complementary therapies for the menopause, *Maturitas*, **66**, 333–343.

Braun, L.A., Tiralongo, E., Wilkinson, J., Spitzer, O., Bailey, M., Poole, S., and Dooley, M. (2010). Perceptions, use and attitudes of pharmacy customers on complementary medicines and pharmacy practice, *BMC Complementary and Alternative Medicine*, **10**, 38.

Brown, W.J., Bryson, L., Byles, J.E., Dobson, A.J., Lee, C., Mishra, G., and Schofield, M. (1998). Women's health Australia: Recruitment for a national longitudinal cohort study, *Women's Health*, **28**, 23–40.

Brown, W.J., Dobson, A.J., Bryson, L., and Byles, J.E. (1999). Women's health Australia: On the progress of the main study cohorts, *Journal of Women's Health and Gender Based Medicine*, **8**, 681–688.

Buick, D.L., Crook, D., and Horne, R. (2005). Women's perceptions of hormone replacement therapy: Risks and benefits (1980–2002). A literature review, *Climacteric*, **8**, 24–35.

Burke, G.L., Legault, C., Anthony, M., Bland, D.R., Morgan, T.M., Naughton, M.J., Leggett, K., Washburn, S.A., and Vitolins, M.Z. (2003). Soy protein and isoflavone effects on vasomotor symptoms in peri- and postmeno-pausal women: The Soy Estrogen Alternative Study, *Menopause*, **10**, 147–153.

Cardini, F., Lesi, G., Lombardo, F., and Van Der Sluijs, C. (2010). The use of complementary and alternative medicine by women experiencing menopausal symptoms in Bologna, *BMC Women's Health*, **10**, 7.

Caspi, O., Koithan, M., and Criddle, M.W. (2004). Alternative medicine or "alternative" patients: A qualitative study of patient-oriented decision-making processes with respect to complementary and alternative medicine, *Medical Decision Making*, **24**, 64–79.

Cheema, D., Coomarasamy, A., and El-Toukhy, T. (2007). Non-hormonal therapy of post-menopausal vasomotor symptoms: A structured evidence-based review, *Archives of Gynecology and Obstetrics*, **276**, 463–9.

Crisafulli, A., Marini, H., Bitto, A., Altavilla, D., Squadrito, G., Romeo, A., Adamo, E. B., Marini, R., D'anna, R., Corrado, F., Bartolone, S., Frisina, N., and Squadrito, F. (2004). Effects of genistein on hot flushes in early post-menopausal women: A randomized, double-blind EPT- and placebo-controlled study, *Menopause*, **11**, 400–404.

Daley, A., Macarthur, C., Mcmanus, R., Stokes-Lampard, H., Wilson, S., Roalfe, A., and Mutrie, N. (2006). Factors associated with the use of complementary medicine and non-pharmacological interventions in symptomatic menopausal women, *Climacteric*, **9**, 336–346.

Eisenberg, D., Kessler, R., Van Rompay, M.I., Kaptchuk, T.J., Wilkey, S.A., Appel, S., and Davis, R.B. (2001). Perceptions about complementary therapies relative to conventional therapies among adults who use both: Results from a national survey, *Annals of Internal Medicine*, **135**, 344–351.

Factor-Litvak, P., Cushmnan, L.F., Kronenberg, F., Wade, C., and Kalmuss, D. (2001). Use of complementary and alternative medicine among women in New York City: A pilot study, *The Journal of Alternative and Complementary Medicine*, **7**, 659–666.

Faure, E.D., Chantre, P., and Mares, P. (2002). Effects of a standardized soy extract on hot flushes: A multicenter, double-blind, randomized, placebo-controlled study, *Menopause*, **9**, 329–334.

Featherstone, C., Godden, D., Selvaraj, S., Emslie, M., and Took-Zozaya, M. (2003). Characteristics associated with reported CAM use in patients attending six GP practices in the Tayside and Grampian regions of Scotland: A survey, *Complementary Therapies in Medicine*, **11**, 168–176.

Goh, L.Y., Vitry, A.I., Semple, S.J., Esterman, A., and Luszcz, M.A. (2009). Self-medication with over-the-counter drugs and complementary medications in South Australia's elderly population, *BMC Complementary and Alternative Medicine*, **9**, 42.

Gokhale, L., Sturdee, D.W., and Parsons, A.D. (2003). The use of food supplements among women attending menopause clinics in the West Midlands, *Journal of the British Menopause Society*, **9**, 32–35.

Gold, E.B., Bair, Y., Zhang, G., Utts, J., Greendale, G.A., Upchurch, D., Chyu, L., Sternfeld, B., and Adler, S. (2007). Cross-sectional analysis of specific complementary and alternative medicine (CAM) use by racial/ethnic group and menopausal status: The Study of Women's Health Across the Nation (SWAN), *Menopause*, **14**, 612–623.

Gollschewski, S., Andereson, D., Skerman, H., and Lyons-Wall, P. (2004). The use of complementary and alternative medications by menopausal women in South East Queensland, *Women's Health Issues*, **14**, 165–171.

Gollschewski, S., Anderson, D., Skerman, H., and Lyons-Wall, P. (2005). Associations between the use of complementary and alternative medications and demographic, health and lifestyle factors in mid-life Australian women, *Climacteric*, **8**, 271–278.

Gollschewski, S., Kitto, S., Anderson, D., and Lyons-Wall, P. (2007). Women's perceptions and beliefs about the use of complementary and alternative medicines during menopause, *Complementary Therapies in Medicine*, **16**, 163–168.

Hari Kaur Khalsa, R.Y.T. (2004). How yoga, meditation, and a yogic lifestyle can help women meet the challenges of perimenopause and menopause, *Sexuality, Reproduction and Menopause*, **2**, 169–175.

Hill-Sakurai, L.E., Muller, J., and Thom, D.H. (2008). Complementary and alternative medicine for menopause: A qualitative analysis of women's decision-making, *Journal of General Internal Medicine*, **23**, 619–622.

Javnbakht, M., Hejazikenari, R., and Ghasemi, M. (2009). Effects of yoga on depression and anxiety of women, *Complementary Therapies in Clinical Practice*, **15**, 102–104.

Knight, D.C., Howes, J.B., Eden, J.A., and Howes, L.G. (2001). Effects on menopausal symptoms and acceptability of isoflavone-containing soy powder dietary supplementation, *Climacteric,* **4**, 13–18.

Lunny, C.A. and Fraser, S.N. (2010). The use of complementary and alternative medicines among a sample of Canadian menopausal-aged women, *Journal of Midwifery and Women's Health*, **55**, 335–343.

MacGregor, C.A., Canney, P.A., Patterson, G., McDonald, R., and Paul, J. (2005). A randomised double-blind controlled trial of oral soy supplements versus placebo for treatment of menopausal symptoms in patients with early breast cancer, *European Journal of Cancer*, **41**, 708–714.

Manocha, R., Semmar, B., and Black, D. (2007). A pilot study of a mental silence form of meditation for women in perimenopause, *Journal of Clinical Psychology in Medical Settings*, **14**, 266–273.

Nahas, E.A., Nahas-Neto, J., Orsatti, F.L., Carvalho, E.P., Oliveira, M.L., and Dias, R. (2007). Efficacy and safety of a soy isoflavone extract in postmenopausal women: A randomized, double-blind, and placebo-controlled study, *Maturitas*, **58**, 249–258.

National Prescribing Service (2010). *National Pharmacist Survey*. Available at: www.nps.org.au [Accessed Sept 2012].

Newton, K.M., Buist, D.S.M., Keenan, N.L., Anderson, L.A., and Lacroix, A.Z. (2002). Use of alternative therapies for menopause symptoms: Results of a population based survey, *Obstetrics and Gynecology*, **100**, 18–25.

Nikander, E., Rutanen, E.M., Nieminen, P., Wahlstrom, T., Ylikorkala, O., and Tiitinen, A. (2005). Lack of effect of isoflavonoids on the vagina and endometrium in postmenopausal women, *Fertility and Sterility*, **83**, 137–142.

Pirotta, M., Kotsirilos, V., Brown, J., Adams, J., Morgan, T., and Williamson, M. (2011). Complementary medicine in general practice — a national survey of GP attitudes and knowledge, *Australian Family Physician*, **39**, 946–950.

Rayner, J.A., McLachlan, H.L., Forster, D.A., and Cramer, R. (2009). Australian women's use of complementary and alternative medicines to enhance fertility: Exploring the experiences of women and practitioners, *BMC Complementary and Alternative Medicine*, **9**, 52.

Rees, R.W., Feigel, I., Vickers, A., Zollman, C., McGurk, R., and Smith, C. (2000). Prevalence of complementary therapy use by women with breast cancer: A population-based survey, *European Journal of Cancer*, **36**, 1359–1364.

Robinson, A. and McGrail, M.R. (2004). Disclosure of CAM use to medical practitioners: A review of qualitative and quantitative studies, *Complementary Therapies in Medicine*, **12**, 90–98.

Rupert, R.L. (2000). A survey of practice patterns and the health promotion and prevention attitudes of US chiropractors. Maintenance Care: Part I, *Journal of Manipulative and Physiological Therapeutics*, **23**, 1–9.

Sayakhot, P., Vincent, A., and Teede, H. (2011). Breast cancer and menopause: Perceptions of diagnosis, menopausal therapies and health behaviours, *Climacteric*, **15**, 59–67.

Scambia, G., Mango, D., Signorile, P.G., Anselmi Angeli, R.A., Palena, C., Gallo, D., Bombardelli, E., Morazzoni, P., Riva, A., and Mancuso, S. (2000). Clinical effects of a standardized soy extract in postmenopausal women: A pilot study, *Menopause*, **7**, 105–111.

Smith, J.M., Sullivan, S.J., and Baxter, G.D. (2009). Massage therapy services for health care: A telephone focus group study of drivers for clients' continued use of services, *Complementary Therapies in Medicine*, **17,** 281–291.

Stankiewicz, M., Smith, C., Alvino, H., and Norman, R. (2007). The use of complementary medicine and therapies by patients attending a reproductive medicine unit in South Australia: A prospective survey, *Australian and New Zealand Journal of Obstetrics and Gynaecology*, **47**, 145–149.

Taylor, K. (2009). Paternalism, participation and partnership: The evolution of patient centeredness in the consultation, *Patient Education and Counselling*, **74**, 150–155.

Upmalis, D.H., Lobo, R., Bradley, L., Warren, M., Cone, F.L., and Lamia, C.A. (2000). Vasomotor symptom relief by soy isoflavone extract tablets in post-menopausal women: A multicenter, double-blind, randomized, placebo-controlled study, *Menopause*, **7**, 236–242.

van der Sluijs, C.P., Bensoussan, A., Liyanage, L., and Shah, S. (2007). Women's health during mid-life survey: The use of complementary and alternative medicine by symptomatic women transitioning through menopause in Sydney, *Menopause*, **14**, 397–403.

Wade, C., Chao, M., Kronenberg, F., Cushman, L., and Kalmuss, D. (2008). Medical pluralism among American Women: Results of a national survey, *Journal of Women's Health*, **17**, 829–840.

Wardle, J. (2010). "Menopause", in Sarris, J. and Wardle, J. (eds.), *Clinical Naturopathy: An Evidence-Based Guide*, Chatswood, Elsevier, pp. 401–419.

Wardle, J., Adams, J., and Lui, C. (2010). A qualitative study of naturopathy in rural practice: A focus upon naturopaths' experiences and perceptions of rural patients and demands for their services, *BMC Health Services Research*, **10**, 185.

Xue, C., Zhang, L., Lin, V., Da Costa, C., and Story, D. (2007). Complementary and alternative medicine use in Australia: Results of a national population based survey in 2005, *Journal of Alternative and Complementary Medicine*, **13**, 643–650.

CHAPTER 2

Complementary and Integrative Medicine, Aging and Chronic Illness: Towards an Interprofessional Approach in Primary Health Care

Kevin D. Willison, Sally Lindsay, Marissa Taylor, Harold Schroeder, and Gavin J. Andrews

2.1 Introduction

A landmark event occurred at the World Health Assembly (WHA) in 1977 when the *Declaration of the Alma-Ata* was endorsed, calling for health care systems to adopt alternative approaches and place a greater priority towards, and improve, primary — first contact — health care delivery (Cueto, 2004; O'Neill *et al.*, 2007). Supporting this declaration was the principle that a majority, rather than a minority, of the world's population should benefit from health care systems. More than 30 years later this call for action and change still resonates, particularly in relation to chronic disease and older people. Although chronic diseases of long duration and slow progression (including asthma, arthritis, cardiovascular disease, hypertension, diabetes, cancers, and musculoskeletal disease) are the leading types of illness in all industrialized countries, and older people the largest group of sufferers (Health Council of Canada, 2005; Frank *et al.*, 2003), varying, and often very low, degrees of support and care exist. Indeed, health care systems worldwide lack sufficient chronic disease management related programs, policies, and resources (including personnel) (Willison *et al.*, 2007).

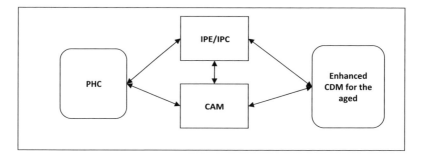

Fig. 2.1   Dialectical strategies to enhance primary health care (PHC) for the aged. Legend: PHC = primary health care; CDM = chronic disease management; CAM = complementary and alternative medicine; IPE/IPC = interprofessional education, interprofessional collaboration.

In the spirit of the Alma-Ata, this chapter considers some alternative directions in care. Although we present a general review of pressing issues, we also aim to be visionary and consider approaches that could be incorporated within primary health care (PHC) settings to initiate or enhance chronic disease management (CDM) efforts (see Fig. 2.1). Specifically we argue that these could include the incorporation of (i) complementary and alternative medicine (CAM) to increase the variety of services provided and to better meet diverse needs and (ii) interprofessional education (IPE) and collaboration (IPC) efforts to stimulate the sharing of expertise between PHC and CAM professionals. We argue that each of these domains might be mutually supportive and bring about improvements within PHC settings. Moreover, we posit that both strategies support the original intent of the *Declaration of the Alma-Ata* and may be feasibly deployed using an integrative medicine approach.

2.2 Understanding Primary Health Care

The Canadian Institute for Health Information (2003) noted that:

> In many ways, primary health care is to the health sector, as the three R's are to education. Just as reading, writing, and arithmetic are fundamental skills that open the door to further learning, primary health care services are the basic tools for health improvement and illness care, and are often

the gateway to other health services (cited in Health Council of Canada, 2005, p. 5).

PHC includes treatment services provided by community-based health professionals, as well as programs that focus upon preventing illness and promoting health. Moreover, PHC services often include referrals to specialists, follow-up, and continuing care of individuals (Shah, 2003). PHC also has the potential for helping to ensure "continuity of care" across health systems which, in turn, is associated with higher patient satisfaction, increased quality of care, and enhanced outcomes (Shortt, 2004).

Although interprofessional PHC exists (including pharmacists, nurse practitioners, midwives, optometrists, dieticians, physiotherapists, and CAM therapists), PHC remains organized predominately around family physicians/general practitioners (GPs), who are "the senior professional group" in terms of management and the leadership of clinical practice (Hutchison *et al.*, 2001). Such arrangements restrict and control the involvement of other health professionals and stifle change and advancement in the system (Gillam, 1999; Shah, 2003). Indeed, according to O'Neill *et al.* (2007), despite a recognized need, there has been a reluctance to tackle the task of reorienting PHC because of the political dominance of biomedicine which is cure-oriented and thereby largely neglects long-term health care (Willison, 1993). Along these lines, Cooper has indicated that:

> The most obvious incongruity between the traditional goals of medicine and the needs of the chronically ill comes from the reality that cure is not a reasonable goal in chronic illness. The goal in chronic illness care is not to restore the patient to optimal health by obliterating the disease, but to maximize the patient's ability to live with the disease. (1990, p. 11)

Thus, as Roth and Harrison (1991) suggest, while the medical model may be appropriate for acute illness, it might be misdirected — even if a still powerful and pervasive force — in the management of chronic illness, and even in understanding the patients' experience of the aging process. An associated critique stresses that biomedicine is limited in part by placing less emphasis upon personal interaction and other social-psychological needs (McCaffrey *et al.*, 2007; Willison, 1993). As such, from a policy perspective there remains a need to reorient the medical profession from its current expensive, clinically based, treatment-focused practice, to a more cost effective system orientated around prevention and ongoing support and care (Willison and Andrews, 2005).

Given the seeming mismatch between the biomedical approach and the care of those with chronic conditions, it is perhaps not surprising that a survey conducted by the Health Council of Canada (2008) found that only half of family physicians studied felt that their practices were well prepared to handle patients with chronic health conditions. This research also found that not all Canadians receive services intended to maintain healthy lifestyles and prevent disease. Only one in five adults reported that their doctors always talked to them about these issues and, an equal number said that their doctors rarely or never did (Health Council of Canada, 2008). Indeed, "for some time, Canadians have been asking for better access to primary health care services, better quality of care, and more health promotion and disease prevention services" (Health Council of Canada, 2008, p. 16).

In sum, an effective PHC system is needed within countries and worldwide that is comprehensive in scope and emphasizes, not only curative needs, but also health promotion, preventative, and rehabilitation services (Public Health in the Public Interest, 2003; Canadian Nurses Association, 2003; Willison et al., 2005a). Incorporating such services could better address the care needs of older people and those with chronic illness. Moreover, such services would provide important foundations for developing chronic disease management programs and strategies.

2.3 The Need to Consider CAM

The Alma-Ata supports the idea that PHC "should be sustained by integrated, functional, and mutually supportive referral systems, leading to the progressive improvement of comprehensive health care for all, and giving priority to those most in need" (O'Neill et al., 2007, p. 5). Moreover, the Alma-Ata supports the goal of providing rehabilitative services within communities. Arguably the integration of regulated forms of CAM within PHC settings has the potential to help meet both of these goals (Adams et al., 2009a).

To this end, PHC providers need to strive to link varied modes of care into single systems, which then provide a range of concurrent, integrated services (Habicht and Berman, 1987; Starfield, 1998). The inclusion of CAM would help achieve certain benchmarks in PHC (specifically, quality, effectiveness, access, continuity, productivity, and responsiveness — Chauvette, 2003). For example, as chronic musculoskeletal pain is a common problem presented to practitioners of PHC (Davies, 1996), access to licensed massage therapists, who are especially trained to treat such conditions, might achieve positive results, both for clients and PHC practices (Sibbritt and Adams, 2010; Willison, 2006a). Indeed, researchers have noted that the content and individualized style and longer consultation times of many CAM modalities can be immensely reassuring, involving close attention to even "trivial" symptoms and signs (King, 1985). In turn, close and longer contact between the therapist and client improves overall client satisfaction. Notably, older people in particular are reported to benefit from, and enjoy, these aspects of CAM, and also from a sense of empowerment with respect to their chronic conditions and care (Adams *et al.*, 2009b; Andrews, 2002).

In terms of integration, current scenarios in health care which include a "meeting point" of some description between conventional and non-conventional approaches are numerous (Adams *et al.*, 2003; Adams, 2004; Adams, 2006; Magin *et al.*, 2006). These might include forms of "structural integration", for example, conventional health professionals in conventional medical environments allowing CAM to be practised by visiting or resident therapists. Otherwise "personal integration" might occur, for example, conventional health professionals in conventional medical environments also practicing CAM themselves. Moreover, some argue that the very idea of integration could be superseded. Singer and Fisher (2007 p. 6) suggest that, "rather than CAM being integrated with biomedicine, a true medical pluralism would allow different beliefs and concepts of health and illness to be endorsed and respected as equals, as occurred before biomedical hegemony". More generally, perpetuating an ongoing debate focused upon which is superior is counter-productive as elements of both CAM and conventional health care offer at least the potential of helping to maintain and/or improve a person's health and/or health-related quality of life (Adams *et al.*, 2009a; Kopec and Willison, 2003).

A key factor which hinders the moving of CAM into mainstream PHC is that of cost. To the general public, the word "complementary" is a misnomer as it can easily be confused as meaning "free". However, CAM services are by no means free and can be expensive to whoever is paying, particularly if required regularly and on an ongoing basis. Unless covered by individual and/or health insurance plans, CAM services are often paid for out-of-pocket in many countries. In turn, the poor and the most vulnerable — who are often older people and those with chronic illness — have limited access to CAM services (Willison *et al.*, 2005a; Willison, 2006a). Moreover, in addition to issues related to access, a range of ethical and moral dilemmas arise with the private CAM sector simultaneously providing care whilst profit making (Andrews *et al.*, 2003).

2.4 Counting the Costs

Due to population aging, chronic disease is a major and increasing cost which, in publicly funded health systems, is and will continue to be passed on to taxpayers. In this context, while there are those who question the cost-effectiveness and financial sustainability of CAM (Kemper *et al.*, 2007), there are others who indicate that there may be cost savings achieved by using CAM interventions, within a variety of clinical settings (Doran *et al.*, 2012; Ford *et al.*, 2010; Solomon *et al.*, 2011; WHCCAM, 2002). For example, a study undertaken by Peru's *National Program in Complementary Medicine* found that traditional (CAM-oriented) treatments were particularly efficacious in treating such pathologies as moderate osteoarthritis, back pain, anxiety disorders, intermittent asthma, peptic ulcer disease, and tension migraines (Fink, 2002). In general, unlike conventional medical care which relies heavily on expensive technology and pharmaceuticals, similar to most PHC settings, CAM exists in a low-tech arena and, therefore, is generally less costly to provide (Sarnat and Winterstein, 2004).

There are also links between CAM and conventional medicine related to costs. CAM users have reported that their use of conventional medical services and prescription drugs decreased after their use of CAM services (Stewart *et al.*, 2001). Furthermore, Sarnat and Winterstein (2004) found that CAM use in conjunction with biomedicine resulted in a decrease in the number of hospital admissions (reduction of 43%), hospital days (reduction of 58.4%), outpatient surgeries and procedures (reduction of 43.2%), as well as pharmaceutical utilization (reduction in cost of 51.8%).

Nevertheless, despite such potential cost savings, there are physicians who have expressed concerns regarding being suitably reimbursed for using CAM. These doctors question whether integrative medicine is profitable (for their practice) claiming that the time-intensive nature of integrative medicine increases the challenge for PHC providers to make a liveable income (Hamre *et al.*, 2006).

2.5 Chronic Disease Management

Primary health care reforms necessary to improve the care of older people and to better address issues related to chronic illness are arguably best framed under CDM strategies and initiatives (Schull, 2005). In terms of approach, CDM is a holistic and comprehensive way of providing health care that emphasizes ways to maintain independence and keep as healthy as possible through the prevention, early detection, and management of chronic conditions. Moreover, it often embodies strategies that offer holistic and comprehensive care, with a focus on rehabilitation (Willison and Andrews, 2005; Willison *et al.*, 2007).

In terms of practice, effective CDM programs educate people with chronic (long-term) conditions on such topics as how to live well and how to take more responsibility for their own care. This is often being pursued in health systems by the development and implementation of self-management workshops providing guidance to clients on such topics as stress management, goal setting, and coping with pain and fatigue. Indeed, the idea is that those with chronic conditions must become partners in their own care as it is they who have the disease or condition, and it is they who have the primary responsibility to manage that disease or condition on a day-to-day basis, in collaboration with their physician and other caregivers (Willison, 2006b). In terms of outcomes, it has been reported that the use of CDM strategies can increase the potential to improve health behaviors (such as exercise), health status as well as life expectancy and quality of life (National Health Service, 2005). Moreover, as a consequence, CDM could also eventually lead to lower health care utilization (Dongbo *et al.*, 2003; Schull, 2005; Wong *et al.*, 2004). The fact that the number of chronically ill people worldwide is increasing — as evident by epidemiological changes within Western societies (Elzen *et al.*, 2007) — is necessitating an expansion of CDM initiatives (Willison *et al.*, 2007; Willison, 2006b; Willison, 2005).

Despite the potential of CDM for health systems, research suggests that an informal form of CDM is currently practised by many older people without health providers having a broad overview of their care. In these circumstances, older people "mix and match" conventional and CAM PHC services to meet their own ends — many times without informing their doctor of their CAM use (Adams *et al.*, 2009b; Andrews, 2002). Whilst empowering, this is far from ideal, raises safety issues, and ultimately may compromise care and health.

2.6 Interprofessional Education and Collaboration

Collaboration between different professional groups is an essential element in the provision of high quality care for people with complex health and social needs such as older people (Fowler *et al.*, 2010). To help pursue this, interprofessional collaboration (IPC) and its corollary interprofessional education (IPE) is recommended. Both aim to improve practice in order to improve outcomes (Stone, 2006).

In general, IPE refers to occasions when two or more professions learn from and about each other to improve collaboration in health and social care. Indeed, IPE involves socializing all health care providers to work together in shared problem solving and decision making, to help bring about and maintain an integrative medical approach (Fowler *et al.*, 2010). In terms of benefits IPE enables people to become "intellectual entrepreneurs" wherein individuals are trained to act responsibly and responsively in the face of multiple and possibly conflicting models of self, others, and the world. IPE aims to foster learning to aid the integration of disparate knowledge structures, such as CAM and biomedicine, into a single action plan. Indeed, Hall *et al.* (2006) advocate that interdisciplinary scholarship requires the deconstruction of knowledge and identity, which may then be reconfigured into new forms of knowledge and action. By doing so, professionals of varied disciplines are better able to manage different value systems, different ways of knowing, plus different ways of acting and relating. Potentially, the establishment of an IPE infrastructure should help stimulate, create, and sustain the type of vibrant environment needed for an integrative medicine (IM) approach to thrive (Cohen, 2004).

A viable outcome of this approach is that CAM practitioners are encouraged not to stereotype the allopathic medical profession as being solely concerned with technology, as failing to be concerned with holistic and preventive care, or as being unresponsive to the full range of patient needs. On the other hand, conventional medical practitioners are encouraged to better understand how forms of CAM may be beneficial and used alongside their practice. In short, IPE helps health care professionals broaden their perspectives beyond their own specialist area. Team working, integration, and workplace flexibility can only be achieved when there is widespread recognition and respect for the specialist base of each profession (Adams *et al.*, 2009a).

A number of barriers and challenges exist with implementing IPE. The first regards professional territories. Not surprisingly, individual health disciplines and medical subspecialties have a sense of ownership regarding their "own" practice and training domains (Tovey and Adams, 2001). In this regard, collaboration between training bodies will be an essential prerequisite to achieving the compromises and changes that will be necessary in curricula and training. The second challenge regards overcoming resistance by organizations and organizational cultures. Organizations have differing structures, operational philosophies, languages, and values, many of which can be entrenched (Fowler *et al.*, 2010; Putnam, 2007). Thus, IPE will need to be implemented differently in different contexts; tailored to suit individual institutions. The third challenge regards the potential dilution of expertise. Of course, IPE should not make health education too generic; the particular skills and expertise that are fundamental to the role that individual health disciplines possess in specific conditions will need to be protected. The fourth is establishing consumer input — such as from older people and those with chronic illness — to ensure that person-centered and preferred care is provided. This alone will be a major challenge to many professional bodies. The fifth and final challenge is measuring outcomes, to find ways to better measure the impact of IPE initiatives (Willison, 2010).

2.7 Conclusion

Pursuits to improve PHC delivery for older people and those with chronic illness must be ongoing. As addressed in this chapter, this could be pursued by incorporating into PHC regulated forms of CAM as well as goals and orientations inherent within an IPE and IPC approach. Indeed, the use of IPE/IPC could lead to an improved interdisciplinary (holistic) approach evoking improvements in the health and well-being of patients, clients, families and communities (Freeth *et al.*, 2005). This alone demands further reflection and research.

Underlying this, an improved dialogue between CAM and PHC professionals is needed. This demands improved reflexivity amongst members of both domains. Instead of continually "measuring each other up" as to what the other's limitations are, focus instead could be on what each other, both separately and collectively, may contribute. While different paths are often taken to a desired end, both CAM and biomedical oriented professionals have important similarities in terms of objectives: namely, the desire to improve the health and well-being of the people they serve. Indeed, this is why many entered health care in the first place. Using this commonality and guidelines, as set out by an IPE approach, both CAM and conventional PHC workers may then move forward together by sharing their knowledge and skills. Doing so will likely not only help build respect for each other, but also and more importantly contribute towards improving patient-centered (holistic) care. Such partnering has the potential to multiply insights and improve creative problem-solving. Collectively, such efforts may help facilitate the original intent as well as long-term and short-term goals embodied within the *Declaration of the Alma-Ata*.

References

Adams, J. (2004). Examining the sites of interface between CAM and conventional health care: Extending the sociological gaze, *Complementary Therapies in Medicine*, **12**, 69–70.

Adams, J. (2006). The use of complementary and alternative medicines within hospital midwifery: Models of care and professional struggle, *Complementary Therapies in Clinical Practice*, **12(1)**, 40–47.

Adams, J., Hollenberg, D., Broom, A., and Lui, C. (2009a). Contextualising integration: A critical social science approach to integrative health care, *Journal of Manipulative and Physiological Therapeutics*, **32(9)**, 792–798.

Adams, J., Lui, C., and McLaughlin, D. (2009b). The use of complementary and alternative medicine in later life, *Expert Reviews in Clinical Gerontology*, **19**, 227–236.

Adams, J., Sibbritt, D., and Easthope, G. (2003). Examining the relationship between women's health and the use of complementary and alternative medicine (CAM), *Complementary Therapies in Medicine*, **11(3)**, 156–158.

Andrews, G.J., Peters, E., and Hammond, R. (2003). Receiving money for medicine: Some tensions and resolutions for community-based private complementary therapists, *Health and Social Care in the Community*, **11(2)**, 155–168.

Andrews, G.L. (2002). Private complementary medicine and older people: Service use and user empowerment, *Ageing and Society*, **22**, 343–368.

Canadian Institute for Health Information (2003). *Health Care in Canada*, CIHI, Toronto.

Canadian Nurses Association (2003). Primary health care — The time has come, *Nursing Now: Issues and Trends in Canadian Nursing*, **16**, 1–4.

Chauvette, M. (2003). *Choices for Change: The Path for Restructuring Primary Healthcare Services in Canada*, Canadian Health Services Research Foundation, Ottawa.

Cohen, M. (2004). CAM practitioners and "regular" doctors: Is integration possible? *Medical Journal of Australia*, **180(12)**, 645–6.

Cohen, M., Ruggie, M., and Micozzi, M.S. (2007). *The Practice of Integrative Medicine: A Legal and Operational Guide*, Springer, New York.

Cooper, M.C. (1990). Chronic illness and nursing's ethical challenge, *Holistic Nursing Practice*, **5(1)**, 10–16.

Cueto, M. (2004). The origins of primary health care and selective primary health care, *American Journal of Public Health*, **94(11)**, 1864–1874.

Davies, A.E. (1996). Primary Care Management of Chronic Musculoskeletal Pain, *The Nurse Practitioner*, **21(8)**, 79–82.

Deng, G. and Cassileth, B.R. (2005). Integrative oncology: Complementary therapies for pain, anxiety, and mood disturbance, *CA: A Cancer Journal for Clinicians*, **55**, 109–116.

Dongbo, F., Hua, F., McGowan, P. Yie, S., Lizhen, Z., Huiqin, Y., Jianguo, M., Shitai, Z., Yongming, D., and Zhihua, W. (2003) Implementation and quantitative evaluation of chronic disease self-management programme in Shanghai, China: Randomized controlled trial, *Bulletin of the World Health Organization*, **81(3)**, 174–182.

Doran, C., Chang, D., Kiat, H., and Bensoussan, A. (2012). "Review of economic methods in complementary and alternative medicine", in Adams, J., Andrews, G., Barnes, Broom, A., and Magin, P. (eds.), *Traditional, Complementary and Integrative Medicine: An International Reader*, Palgrave, London.

Elzen, H., Slaets, J.P.G., Snijders, T.A.B., and Steverink, N. (2007). Evaluation of the chronic disease self-management program (CDSMP) among chronically ill older people in the Netherlands, *Social Science and Medicine*, **64**, 1832–1841.

Fink, S. (2002). International efforts spotlight traditional complementary and alternative medicine, *American Journal of Public Health*, **92(11)**, 1734–1739.

Ford, E., Solomon, D., Adams, J., and Graves, N. (2010). The use of economic evaluation in CAM: An introductory framework, *BMC Complementary and Alternative Medicine*, 10, 66.

Fowler, P., Hannigan, B., and Northway, R. (2010). Community nurses and social workers learning together: A report of an interprofessional education initiative in South Wales, *Health and Social Care in the Community*, **8(3)**, 186–191.

Frank, J., Ruggiero, E.D., and Moloughney, B. (2003). *The Future of Public Health in Canada: Developing a Public Health System for the 21st Century. Canadian Institutes of Health Research, Executive Summary*, Government of Canada, Ad Hoc Committee on the Future of Public Health in Canada, Ottawa.

Freeth, D., Hammick, M., Reeves, S., Koppel, I., and Barr, H. (2005). *Effective Interprofessional Education: Development, Delivery and Evaluation*, Blackwell, Oxford.

Gillam, S. (1999) A public health model of primary care: From concept to reality. Book review, *Family Practice*, **16(2)**, 209–210.

Habicht, J.-B. and Berman, P.A. (1987). Editorial — Strategies in primary health care, *American Journal of Public Health*, **77(11)**, 1396–1397.

Hall, J.G., Bainbridge, L., Buchan, A., Cribb, A., Drummond, J., Gyles, C., Hicks, T.P., McWilliam, C., Paterson, B., Ratner, P.A., Skarakis-Doyle, E., and Solomon, P. (2006). A meeting of minds: Interdisciplinary research in the health sciences in Canada, *Canadian Medical Association Journal*, **175(7)**, 763–768.

Hamre, H., Witt, C., Glockmann, A., Troger, W., Willich, S., and Kiene, H. (2006). Use and safety of anthroposophic medications in chronic disease: A 2-year prospective analysis, *Drug Safety*, **29(12)**, 1173–89.

Health Council of Canada (2005). *Primary Health Care*. Available online: http:// healthcouncilcanada.ca [Accessed Nov 2011].

Health Council of Canada (2008). *Fixing the Foundation: An Update on Primary Health Care and Home Care Renewal in Canada*. Available online: http:// healthcouncilcanada.ca [Accessed Nov 2011].

Hutchison, B., Abelson, J., and Lavis, J. (2001). Primary care in Canada: So much innovation, so little change, *Health Affairs*, **20(3)**, 116–131.

Kemper, K., Dirkse, D., Eadie, D., and Pennington, M. (2007). What do clinicians want? Interest in integrative health services at a North Carolina academic medical center, *BMC Complementary & Alternative Medicine*, **7**, 5.

Kendall, D. (2007). *Sociology in Our Times: The Essentials*, Wadsworth, Belmont.

King, K. (1985). Alternative medicine, *Medical Journal of Australia*, **142(10)**, 547–550.

Kopec, J. and Willison, K.D. (2003). A comparative review of four preference-weighted measures of health-related quality of life, *Journal of Clinical Epidemiology*, **56(4)**, 317–325.

Lumague, M., Morgan, A., Mak, D., Hanna, M., Kwong, J., Cameron, C., Zener, D., and Sinclair, L. (2006). Interprofessional education: The student perspective, *Journal of Interprofessional Care*, **20(3)**, 246–253.

Magin, P., Adams, J., Heading, G., Pond, D., and Smith, W. (2006). Complementary and alternative medicine therapies in acne, psoriasis and atopic eczema: Results of a qualitative study of patients' experiences and perceptions, *Journal of Alternative and Complementary Medicine*, **12(5)**, 451–457.

McCaffrey, A.M., Pugh, G.F., and O'Conner, B.B. (2007). Understanding patient preferences for integrative medical care: Results from patient focus groups, *Journal of General Internal Medicine*, **22(11)**, 1500–1505.

National Health Service (2005). *Self Care — A Real Choice*, DH Publications, London.

O'Neill, M., Dupéré, S., Pederson, A., and Rootman, I. (2007). *Health Promotion in Canada: Critical Perspectives*, Canadian Scholars' Press, Toronto.

Public Health in the Public Interest (2003). *The Canadian Coalition for Public Health in the 21st Century, Brief to the Senate Committee on Social Affairs, Science and Technology*, October 2003.

Putnam, M. (2007). *Aging and Disability: Crossing Network Lines*, Springer, New York.

Roth, P.A. and Harrison, J.K. (1991). Orchestrating social change: An imperative in care of the chronically ill, *Journal of Medicine and Philosophy*, **16(3)**, 343–359.

Saks, M. (2000). "Professionalization, politics and CAM", in Kelner, M., Wellman, B., Pescosolido B., and Saks, M. (eds.), *Complementary and Alternative Medicine: Challenge and Change*, Harwood, Amsterdam, pp. 223–238.

Sarnat, R.L. and Winterstein, J. (2004). Clinical and cost outcomes of an integrative medicine IPA, *Journal of Manipulative and Physiological Therapeutics*, **27(5)**, 336–347.

Schull, M.J. (2005). Rising utilization of US emergency departments: Maybe it's time to stop blaming the patients, *Annals of Emergency Medicine*, **45(1)**, 13–14.

Shah, C. (2003). *Public Health and Preventative Medicine in Canada*, Elsevier, Canada.

Shortt, S.E.D. (2004). "Primary care reform: Is there a clinical rational?", in Wilson, R., Shortt, S.E.D., and Dorland, J. (eds.), *Implementing Primary Care Reform: Barriers and Facilitators*, McGill-Queen's University Press, Kingston, pp. 11–24.

Sibbritt, D. and Adams, J. (2009). Back pain amongst 8,910 young Australian women: A longitudinal analysis of the use of conventional providers, complementary and alternative medicine (CAM) providers and self-prescribed CAM, *Clinical Rheumatology*, **29**, 25–32.

Singer, J. and Fisher, K. (2007). The impact of co-option on herbalism: A bifurcation in epistemology and practice, *Health Sociology Review*, **16 (1)**, 18–26.

Solomon, D., Ford, E., Adams, J., and Graves, N. (2011). The potential of St John's Wort for the treatment of depression. The economic perspective, *Australian and New Zealand Journal of Psychiatry*, **45(2)**, 123–130.

Starfield, B. (1998). *Primary Care: Balancing Health Needs, Services and Technology*, Oxford University Press, Oxford.

Stewart, D., Weeks, J., and Bent, S. (2001). Utilization, patient satisfaction and cost implications of acupuncture, massage, and naturopathic medicine offered as covered health benefits: A comparison of two delivery methods, *Alternative Therapies*, **7(4)**, 66–70.

Stone, N. (2006). Evaluating interprofessional education: The tautological need for interdisciplinary approaches, *Journal of Interprofessional Care*, **20(3)**, 260–275.

Tovey, P. and Adams, J. (2001). Primary care as intersecting social worlds, *Social Science and Medicine*, **52**, 695–706.

WHCCAM (2002). *White House Commission on Complementary and Alternative Medicine Policy. Final Report*. Available at: www.whccamp.hhs.gov/fr7.html [Accessed Nov 2011].

WHO (2002). *WHO Traditional Medicine Strategy 2002–2005*. World Health Organization, Geneva.

Willison, K.D. (2010). Enhancing validity of multidisciplinary learning assessment tools. Reaching potential: Assessment as a transformative process. Educational Conference, 30 April 2010. Wilfrid Laurier University, Waterloo, Ontario, Canada.

Willison, K.D. (2006a). Integrating Swedish massage therapy with primary health care initiatives as part of a holistic nursing approach, *Complementary Therapies in Medicine*, **14(4)**, 254–260.

Willison, K.D. (2005). Linking massage therapy to public health and primary health care initiatives, *Massage Therapy Canada*, **Fall**, 31.

Willison, K.D. (2006b). *Promoting Self-Care and Chronic Disease Management through Community Based Research*, Ontario Health Promotion E-Bulletin (OHPE). Available at: http://www.ohpe.ca/index.php?option=com_content&task=view&id=7747&Itemid=78 [Accessed Nov 2011].

Willison, K.D. (1993). *The Care of the Chronically-Ill Elderly Patient in an Acute Care Hospital in Light of the Biomedical Science Approach*. Unpublished Master of Arts Thesis, available via the Department of Sociology, Lakehead University, Thunder Bay, Ontario, Canada.

Willison, K.D. and Andrews, G.J. (2004). Complementary medicine and older people: Past research and future directions, *Complementary Therapies in Nursing and Midwifery*, **10(2)**, 80–91.

Willison, K.D. and Andrews, G.J. (2005). The potential of public health to enhance chronic disease management, *Public Health*, **119(12)**, 1130–1132.

Willison, K.D., Andrews, G.J., and Cockerham, W.C. (2005a). Life chance characteristics of older Swedish massage therapy users and former users, *Complementary Therapies in Clinical Practice*, **11(4)**, 232–241.

Willison, K.D., Williams, P., and Andrews, G.J. (2007). Enhancing chronic disease management: A review of key issues and strategies, *Complementary Therapies in Clinical Practice*, **13**, 232–239.

Wong, J, Gilbert, J., and Kilburn, L. (2004). *Seeking Program Sustainability in Chronic Disease Management: The Ontario Experience*, The Change Foundation, Toronto.

CHAPTER 3

Complementary and Alternative Medicine and Skin Disease in General Practice

Parker Magin and Jon Adams

3.1 Introduction

Skin disease is common in general practice and recent work shows 16.8% of general practice consultations in Australia dealt with a skin disease (Britt *et al.*, 2011). In this chapter we explore the relationship between general practice, CAM, and skin disease. Initially the chapter provides an overview of CAM therapies as used by patients with skin conditions. We then address the prevalence of CAM use for skin disease in different clinical and non-clinical contexts (including general practice) before more closely examining the relationship of GPs (CAM-practising or CAM-advocating, and those antipathetic to CAM) with CAM use in skin diseases. Central to these CAM-GP relationships are issues around evidence of efficacy, adverse effects, quality control, and ethics. These issues will be illustrated with the example of atopic eczema, a common skin disorder for which many CAM therapies have been advocated and for which CAM therapies are most commonly used.

3.2 CAM and the Skin

Population-based studies have shown those with skin disease are more likely to be CAM users than those without skin disease (Birdee *et al.*,

2010). CAM therapies have a particular role in the management of skin diseases. Intrinsic characteristics and clinical features of common skin diseases and the demographics of those who suffer from skin disease may contribute to this. CAM therapies are especially used in chronic medical conditions (Bausell *et al.*, 2001; Williams *et al.*, 2011), and chronic diseases are particularly common in dermatological practice (Hong *et al.*, 2008). Much CAM therapy is self-accessed rather than prescribed by a CAM or allopathic medicine practitioner (Eisenberg *et al.*, 1998), and much skin disease is perceived as being less medically important than "life-threatening" conditions — sometimes by doctors and even by some patients with skin disease (Magin *et al.*, 2009). An inference might then be that many circumstances of skin disease are quite appropriately self-managed and that CAM therapies may be a viable option for skin disease sufferers in the self-management of their condition. A further factor to consider in terms of examining the relationship of CAM and skin disease is that the age at first use of CAM is decreasing (Kessler *et al.*, 2001). Many of the most common skin diseases characteristically have their onset in infancy or childhood (atopic eczema) or in adolescence (acne). This may have particular implications for adverse effects profiles and for ethical considerations of CAM use in skin disease. This will be discussed later in this chapter.

3.2.1 *Which CAM therapies are used in skin diseases?*

The provenance of CAM therapies from across a range of disparate disciplines, and their being often non-regulated and often self-accessed, makes comprehensive surveys of practice inherently difficult. As such, the range of CAM therapies employed in skin diseases (themselves a broad and heterogeneous grouping of conditions) is difficult to document. Categorising CAM therapies used in skin diseases constitutes a formidable challenge — in both number and diversity of CAM therapies. A comprehensive digest is thus beyond the scope of this chapter, but the extent of usage can be illustrated by the example of acne vulgaris (the most prevalent of all the skin diseases). A recent overview (not comprehensive) of some of the CAM therapies cited in the literature as being used in acne (Magin *et al.*, 2006b) identified 27 essential oils, 26 topical herbs or plants, five ingested herbs or plants, three homeopathic medicines, four topical Asian therapies, and six topical or ingested inhibitors of 5-alpha reductase, as well as Indian Ayurvedic therapies, acupuncture, blood-letting, skin pricking, cupping, and various other miscellaneous treatments (Magin *et al.*, 2006b).

In 2002 (Smith *et al.*, 2009) and 2007 (Fuhrmann *et al.*, 2009) the alternative health supplement of the National Health Interview Survey provided an opportunity to investigate CAM modalities used for skin diseases in the United States. Those most used were vitamins and minerals, herbal supplements, homeopathy, acupuncture, and relaxation. These results, however, should be interpreted with caution as the absolute numbers of respondents using CAM specifically for skin disease were small and, as the authors note, ascertainment of those with true skin disease in self-report surveys is difficult (Fuhrmann *et al.*, 2009). In studies of British, Taiwanese, Singaporean, and Israeli dermatology outpatients, the most commonly used modalities have been herbal therapies, homeopathy, dietary therapies, traditional Chinese medicine, acupuncture, and Indian traditional medicine. Aromatherapy, acupuncture, hypnotherapy, reflexology, and massage use have also been identified (Baron *et al.*, 2005; Ben-Arye *et al.*, 2003; Johnston *et al.*, 2003; Nicolaou and Johnston, 2004; Lee *et al.*, 2004).

3.2.2 *CAM use: which skin diseases?*

The most common skin diseases for which CAM was used among participants in studies of British and Turkish skin disease patients (Gonul *et al.*, 2009) and patients in a National Health Service facility dedicated to CAM (Sharples *et al.*, 2003) were psoriasis, eczema/dermatitis, and acne. Documentation of CAM therapies employed in the treatment of skin diseases is best seen for the three most common dermatological conditions — psoriasis (Ben-Arye *et al.*, 2003; Fleischer *et al.*, 1996; Magin *et al.*, 2006a; Jensen, 1990), atopic eczema (Lee and Bielory, 2010, Johnston *et al.*, 2003, Magin *et al.*, 2006a, Jensen, 1990) and acne (Yarnell and Abascal, 2006; Magin *et al.*, 2006a, 2006b). But the range of skin diseases for which use of CAM has been documented is wide. Warts, urticaria and fungal skin infections are other examples of common skin conditions for which use of CAM therapies has been noted (Gonul *et al.*, 2009). Even skin malignancies have been documented as having been treated with CAM — 14% of melanoma patients at an Austrian university melanoma clinic admitted use of CAM therapies for their melanoma (Sollner *et al.*, 1997).

Of additional note is that beyond these disease-specific uses of CAM therapies there is a range of CAM usage that is not dependent on dermatological disease nosologies. In these instances CAM is used for non-disease-specific indications. Some self-accessed CAM skin products are used "generically" by some individuals — that is, used for any skin condition or any manifestation of disordered skin (Magin *et al.*, 2006a). It has been noted (Magin *et al.*, 2006b) that in an ethnopharmacognostic survey of an Italian region (Pieroni *et al.*, 2004) a large number of phytotherapies were used for non-disease-specific purposes rather than for defined skin diseases. Particular CAM therapies were used for reddened or inflamed skin, as a facial "skin toner" or skin-cleanser, to "smooth" facial skin, or to treat "sores" or "rashes". A philosophical construct underlying this finding and previously observed by Dattner (2003), is that many CAM or traditional therapeutic systems "have cosmologies for choosing herbs which are based on the characteristics of the given patient" rather than on the disease or pathological process underlying their presentation.

Even in cultures where allopathic medicine is the established "mainstream" of health care, CAM use may not reflect the medical paradigm of specific treatment of a defined and diagnosed disease entity. In a United States population it was noted that among those with skin disease who used CAM therapies the most common reason for using CAM was not treatment of the specific skin condition but was for "general wellness or disease prevention" (Fuhrmann *et al.*, 2009).

3.3 Prevalence of CAM use for Skin Diseases

The prevalence of CAM use for skin conditions has been examined in dermatological populations, in general medical populations, in populations of CAM-users, and in general population samples.

3.3.1 *Prevalence of CAM use in clinical settings: dermatology and general practice populations*

A number of studies have examined the relationship of skin disease and CAM in specialist dermatology settings. Based upon international studies of dermatology outpatients between 15% and 35% of patients have been reported as treating their skin disease with CAM therapies (See *et al.*, 2011; Gonul *et al.*, 2009). Of dermatology outpatients with psoriasis, an Israeli study showed that 45.8% were using or had used CAM therapies in the past year (Ben-Arye *et al.*, 2003) and in a United States study 51% were using CAM (Fleischer *et al.*, 1996). For atopic eczema, a study of an English paediatric outpatients clinic reported 46% of patients had used or were currently using, and a further 17% intended to use, CAM therapies (Johnston *et al.*, 2003). A study of CAM use for contact dermatitis in an English dermatology outpatients clinic reported prevalence of CAM use as being 10% (Nicolaou and Johnston, 2004).

Examining the prevalence of CAM for skin disease among those who use CAM, 14% of patients attending a United Kingdom National Health Service CAM clinic did so for skin conditions (Sharples *et al.*, 2003). Of the 19% of the unselected general practice patients who had used CAM in an Israeli study, 6.5% did so for skin diseases (Kitai *et al.*, 1998). But this was in a relatively small sample taken from only two practices. More meaningful findings have come from community-based general population samples.

3.3.2 *Prevalence of CAM use for skin disease in non-clinical settings: general population samples*

In a moderately-sized (2,055 participants), nationally representative, United States population surveyed in 1997, 8.6% reported having skin disease and 6.7% of this group reported having used CAM for their skin disease in the past 12 months and 2.2% of them had consulted an alternative practitioner for their condition (Eisenberg *et al.*, 1998).

Of two larger (31,044 and 23,393 participants, respectively) nationally representative, United States populations surveyed in 2002 (Smith *et al.*,

2009) and 2007 (Fuhrmann *et al.*, 2009), 8.4% and 10.1%, respectively, reported having skin disease and, of these groups, 2.1% and 1.2%, respectively, reported having used CAM for their skin disease in the previous 12 months.

3.3.3 *Why the differences in prevalence of CAM use for skin disease in clinical versus general population samples?*

From these study findings outlined above it can be seen that there is a much lower prevalence of CAM use for skin disease among those sampled from the general population (who have skin disease) when compared to those sampled from specialist dermatology outpatient populations. It seems that general population prevalence of use is also lower (though less markedly so) than that in general practice samples. This suggests that CAM therapies may tend to be used for the more severe spectrum of skin diseases.

It may be that this, in part, also reflects help-seeking behaviour (for both CAM and allopathic treatments) on the part of some patients with skin disease. It is a finding of a number of studies that patients using CAM also tend to seek allopathic medical care for their skin disease. In a United States population survey (Fuhrmann *et al.*, 2009), 51.5% of participants using CAM for their skin disease also discussed CAM use with a conventional medicine professional. In a qualitative study of patients with acne, psoriasis and atopic eczema (Magin *et al.*, 2006a), those with psoriasis and atopic eczema (chronic, incurable, and often difficult to treat conditions) often adopted an approach to their disease of "try everything under the sun" and practised a "cycling of therapies" (allopathic and CAM) in a desperate attempt to find relief from their disease.

3.4 CAM, Skin Disease and Evidence

Trials of CAM therapies have been criticised for their lack of methodological rigour (Linde *et al.*, 2001). Some CAM disciplines such as homeopathy and therapeutic touch have been criticised as being founded on a rationale that "violates fundamental scientific laws" (Angell and Kassirer,

1998). Angell and Kassirer further criticise alternative medicine as largely ignoring biological mechanisms, and herbal remedies as often sold without any knowledge of their mechanism of action (Angell and Kassirer, 1998). In fact, while convincing empirical evidence of clinical efficacy for CAM in skin diseases may be sparse, there is considerable evidence of biological plausibility for a number of CAM skin therapies.

3.4.1 *Proposed mechanisms of actions for CAM in skin disease*

There is an extensive and expanding evidence base for the pharmacological properties of a great many CAM therapies (Magin and Adams, 2007). This is especially so for phytotherapies. Many studies address the basic mechanisms that underlie disorders of the skin. Thus, multiple CAM therapies used to treat skin complaints have been found, *in vitro* and *in vivo*, to be anti-inflammatory (Magin *et al.*, 2006b; Jellinek and Maloney, 2005), anti-bacterial (Magin *et al.*, 2006b; Farag *et al.*, 2004), anti-fungal (Farag *et al.*, 2004; Zamilpa *et al.*, 2002; Giordani *et al.*, 2004), anti-viral (Farag *et al.*, 2004), anti-androgenic (Magin *et al.*, 2006b), anti-oxidant (Jellinek and Maloney, 2005), anti-carcinogenic (Jellinek and Maloney, 2005), and to reduce the comedogenicity of sebum (Magin *et al.*, 2006b).

In contrast to the extensive literature on the biological attributes of CAM skin therapies, there is a limited literature on their clinical efficacy. We will now consider evidence for CAM therapies in skin diseases, using atopic eczema as our particular example.

3.4.2 *CAM in atopic eczema: evidence for efficacy*

A study eliciting UK GPs' opinions regarding "effectiveness gaps" — areas of clinical practice in which available treatments are not fully effective (see Chapter 8 of this collection for further discussion) — found eczema to be the third most commonly cited condition (after musculoskeletal disorders and depression) (Fisher *et al.*, 2004). Atopic dermatitis is also one of the skin conditions most frequently treated with CAM (Ernst *et al.*, 2002). However, despite the fact that more research has been conducted for CAM in atopic eczema than has been the case for other dermatological conditions, the empirical evidence for such use remains patchy. This research includes trials of medicinal herbs, hypnotherapy, dietary exclusions, relaxation training and other psychological interventions, and probiotics.

Despite some encouraging individual studies, overall results have been contradictory with considerable heterogeneity of results for individual treatments and methodological limitations of positive studies. Convincing evidence of efficacy for any of the CAM treatments in atopic eczema remains frustratingly elusive (Lee and Bielory, 2010; Hoare *et al.*, 2000; Boyle *et al.*, 2009; Zhang *et al.*, 2004; Ernst *et al.*, 2002).

Randomised and non-randomised trials have suggested that traditional Chinese oral herbal preparations are efficacious in atopic eczema (Sheehan *et al.*, 1995; Sheehan and Atherton, 1994; Sheehan *et al.*, 1992; Henderson *et al.*, 2000). But methodological issues with these studies (Zhang *et al.*, 2004), as well as a subsequent negative study (Fung *et al.*, 1999) and unsupportive systematic reviews (Zhang *et al.*, 2004) suggest the issue is not resolved and that the use of Chinese herbal preparations for atopic eczema cannot be recommended without further evidence. Studies subsequent to these systematic reviews do not clarify the situation. A study (with methodological limitations) employing a different preparation, a tri-herbal combination, showed no difference between active preparation and placebo (Shapira *et al.*, 2005) and, in a study in children using a further concoction of an ancestral formula containing five herbs, there was an improvement in quality of life but not of objective eczema severity (Hon *et al.*, 2007).

Dietary supplements of essential fatty acids have been investigated quite intensively in atopic eczema due to their role in epidermal skin barrier function and T cell functioning. But despite initial positive studies reflected in an early systematic review finding evidence for efficacy (Morse *et al.*, 1989), a subsequent systematic review including results from studies of supplements such as evening primrose oil (oral and topical), borage oil, blackcurrent seed oil (all sources of γ-linolenic acid), and fish oils failed to find convincing evidence of clinical efficacy (van Gool *et al.*, 2004; Hoare *et al.*, 2000). A study of infants at risk of atopic eczema (and which included maternal dietary γ-linolenic acid supplementation of breast-fed infants) also failed to show a decrease in the development of atopic eczema (Kitz *et al.*, 2006).

Probiotics have been increasingly used in atopic dermatitis. Probiotics appear to have a favourable risk profile (Kukkonen *et al.*, 2008). Perinatal administration of the probiotic *Lactobacillus rhamnosus* was found to reduce incidence of atopic eczema in at-risk children during the first two years of life, an effect persisting at four years (Kalliomaki *et al.*, 2003). Further studies have had conflicting results (Kuitunen *et al.*, 2009). In terms of treatment of atopic eczema in infants and older children, trials have had inconsistent results. Effect sizes in some of the studies suggest statistically significant findings may be of marginal or modest clinical significance (Boyle and Tang, 2006). Meanwhile, other trials may have lacked statistical power (Boyle and Tang, 2006). Differences in probiotic species and strains also make interpretation of the literature (and clinical application of the findings) problematic. But, overall, a Cochrane review has found that there is no convincing evidence of efficacy (Boyle *et al.*, 2009).

Among other CAM therapies, there is limited evidence for the use of a topical honey/beeswax/olive oil, *Olea europaea,* preparation (Al-Waili, 2003), massage (Schachner *et al.*, 1998), and oolong tea (Uehara *et al.*, 2001) in atopic eczema. Autologous blood transfusion has shown benefit in a single trial (Pittler *et al.*, 2003).

Psychological interventions have been found to be of possible benefit in the treatment of the skin manifestations of atopic eczema (Chida *et al.*, 2007). Autogenic training as a form of relaxation therapy, and cognitive-behavioural treatment were efficacious in a randomised trial (Ehlers *et al.*, 1995), though the positive effect of a psycho-educational stress management program in another study was not significantly better than control. Hypnotherapy has some limited evidence of efficacy (Stewart and Thomas, 1995).

3.5 Adverse Effects of CAM Skin Therapies

As with evidence for clinical efficacy, the lack of systematic monitoring of toxicity or adverse effects of CAM dermatological therapies is problematic for GPs. And, far from being harmless, CAM dermatological therapies have been associated with such adverse effects as contact dermatitis (Ernst, 2000; de Medeiros *et al.*, 2008; Ventura *et al.*, 2006), phytophotodermatitis (Ventura *et al.*, 2006) Stevens–Johnson syndrome (Monk, 1986), photosensitisation (Ernst, 2000), morbilliform rashes (Gelfand *et al.*, 2005), bullous reactions (Gelfand *et al.*, 2005) irritation/dermatitis (Ernst, 2000; Bassett *et al.*, 1990; Morris *et al.*, 2003), and neurotoxicity with coma (Morris *et al.*, 2003). Drawing again upon the example of atopic eczema, we here illustrate demonstrated adverse effects of CAM therapies in skin disease management.

3.5.1 *Adverse effects of CAM therapies used in atopic eczema*

While probiotics have been demonstrated to have very low risk of adverse effects (Kukkonen *et al.*, 2008), this is not so for another of the most commonly documented atopic eczema CAM therapies, Chinese herbal medicines (Graham-Brown, 2000). These have been associated with dilated cardiomyopathy (Ferguson *et al.*, 1997), hepatotoxicity (Sheehan and Atherton, 1994; Ernst, 2000; Verucchi *et al.*, 2002), nephrotoxicity (Lord *et al.*, 1999) and urothelial malignancy (Lord *et al.*, 2001). These toxicities are anecdotal. The issue for GPs is that with few clinical trials to quantify potential adverse effects and, unlike allopathic pharmaceuticals, with no systematic means of recording adverse events of marketed drugs (Choonara, 2003), they are unable to make considered risk-benefit analyses for use of CAM therapies used in atopic eczema.

A further problem for GPs recommending CAM therapies for atopic eczema is the issue of adulteration of CAM therapies. This is well documented for a number of atopic eczema CAM therapies. Ramsay *et al.* (2003) analysed 24 "herbal creams" reported to be efficacious in the treatment of childhood eczema. Twenty of the twenty-four creams contained corticosteroids: clobetasol proprionate, clobetasone butyrate, betamethasone valerate, and hydrocortisone (Ramsay *et al.*, 2003). In a similar study, eight of eleven herbal eczema creams contained dexamethasone (Keane *et al.*, 1999). This adulteration is illegal and can cause permanent skin damage (Daniels *et al.*, 2002).

3.6 Ethical Dimensions of CAM use for Skin Disease in General Practice

In the absence of convincing empirical evidence for CAM therapies in skin disease, and given the demonstrated potential for adverse effects of commonly used CAM skin therapies, GPs may feel that there are ethical constraints on their recommendation of CAM skin therapies for their patients. This may be especially so for their paediatric patients, as much CAM use in skin disease is of childhood atopic eczema. Ethical issues extend beyond recommendation of CAM to acquiescence in patient decisions regarding CAM use — "giving tacit approval to an irresponsible decision" (Adams *et al.*, 2002). Not only might some CAM skin disease therapies entail risk of adverse side effects non-commensurate with their demonstrated efficacy, but "dermatological patients using CAM may also harbour unrealistic expectations regarding CAM" (See *et al.*, 2011) resulting in delaying or failing to diagnose potentially treatable disease and/or failure to access or adhere to efficacious allopathic treatments. It has been suggested that use or recommendation by conventional medical practitioners of CAM therapies lacking scientific evidence or which are beyond the usual practice of the profession may contravene the standards of ethical practice of their professional bodies (Thorne *et al.*, 2002). This is a complex issue. Ethical imperatives of beneficence and nonmaleficence may not be in accord with the principle of respect for the patient's autonomy. Adams *et al.* (2002) identify a potential for serious physician–patient conflict when CAM and conventional medical therapies interact. They also note that the potential for conflict (including physician withdrawal from care) is more acute when the physician involved is the patient's primary care provider and where there is a longitudinal care commitment between physician and patient (Adams *et al.*, 2002). Hence, ethical issues around CAM use by their patients are especially difficult for GPs — often being more problematic than for their specialist colleagues.

The ethical issues for physicians in the problematic area of children's CAM use are particularly relevant for atopic eczema, with its propensity to commence in infancy. Some researchers argue that safety and efficacy are relative and must be interpreted in light of a child's health status and the beliefs, values, and preferences of the wider family unit (Vohra and Cohen,

2007). They suggest that an ethical approach to the paediatric use of CAM demands open communication between families and all their health care providers. With regards to adult CAM use, commentators also advocate communication, suggesting physicians engage in problem-solving with their patients in line with the patient's core values and propose a framework for risk-benefit analysis in decision-making around CAM use for which no reliable evidence exists (Adams *et al.*, 2002).

This framework includes consideration of the illness (severity and acuteness, and curability with conventional medicine), the allopathic treatment (efficacy and adverse effects), the CAM treatment (quality of evidence of safety and efficacy) and the patient (understanding of the risks and benefits of CAM therapy, and acceptance of those risks, and persistence of intent to use CAM) (Adams *et al.*, 2002). Thus, with many skin diseases (psoriasis and atopic eczema, for example) their chronicity and incurability must figure in ethical considerations along with their non-life-threatening nature (although, due to their visibility, skin diseases can be life-ruining (Koo and Lebwohl, 2001)). This risk-benefit framework also assumes some judgement of the quality of the evidence for a given CAM therapy. This, however, may be contentious given current dispute regarding what constitutes appropriate evidence for a range of CAM modalities (Oguamanam, 2006).

3.7 Conclusion

The use of CAM therapies in skin disease is well established, with a wide range of therapies employed in many skin diseases, notably atopic eczema, psoriasis, and acne. There is strong evidence of biological plausibility, though not clinical efficacy, for some CAM therapies used in skin diseases. Thus, CAM therapies, despite the often lack of convincing evidence around clinical efficacy and concerns regarding potential adverse effects and adulteration, may constitute an untapped (in allopathic practice) therapeutic resource in an area where allopathic management faces considerable limitations. Faced with these circumstances, GPs appear to be in an ambivalent position with regard to CAM use in their skin patients and display a range of attitudes and practices with regard to the various CAM modalities used in skin diseases.

References

Adams, K.E., Cohen, M.H., Eisenberg, D., and Jonsen, A.R. (2002). Ethical considerations of complementary and alternative medical therapies in conventional medical settings, *Annals of Internal Medicine*, **137**, 660–664.

Al-Waili, N.S. (2003). Topical application of natural honey, beeswax andolive oil mixture for atopic dermatitis or psoriasis: Partially controlled, single-blinded study, *Complementary Therapies in Medicine*, **11**, 226–234.

Angell, M. and Kassirer, J.P. (1998). Alternative medicine: The risks of untested and unregulated remedies, *New England Journal of Medicine*, **339**, 839–841.

Baron, S.E., Goodwin, R.G., Nicolau, N., Blackford, S., and Goulden, V. (2005). Use of complementary medicine among outpatients with dermatologic conditions within Yorkshire and South Wales, United Kingdom, *Journal of American Academy of Dermatology*, **52**, 589–594.

Bassett, I.B., Pannowitz, D.L., and Barnetson, R.S. (1990). A comparative study of tea-tree oil versus benzoylperoxide in the treatment of acne, *Medical Journal of Australia*, **153**, 455–458.

Bausell, R.B., Lee W.L., and Berman, B.M. (2001). Demographic and health-related correlates to visits to complementary and alternative medical providers, *Medical Care*, **39**, 190–196.

Ben-Arye, E., Ziv, M., and Frenkel, M. (2003). Complementary medicine and psoriasis: linking the patient's outlook with evidence-based medicine, *Dermatology*, **207**, 302–307.

Birdee, G.S., Phillips, R.S., and Davis, R.B. (2010). Factors associated with pediatric use of complementary and alternative medicine, *Pediatrics*, **125**, 249–256.

Boyle, R.J., Bath-Hextall, F.J., and Leonardi-Bee, J. (2009). Probiotics for the treatment of eczema: A systematic review, *Clinical and Experimental Allergy*, **39**, 1117–1127.

Boyle, R.J. and Tang, M.L. (2006). The role of probiotics in the management of allergic disease, *Clinical and Experimental Allergy*, **36**, 568–576.

Britt, H., Miller, G., Charles, J., Henderson, J., Bayram, C., Pan, Y., Valenti, L., Harrison, C., O'Halloran, J., Zhang, C., and Fahridin, S.S. (2011), *General Practice Activity in Australia 2010–11. General Practice Series No. 29*, Sydney University Press, Sydney.

Chida, Y., Steptoe, A., Horakawa, N., Sudo, N., and Kubo, C. (2007). The effects of psychological intervention on atopic dermatitis. A systematic review and meta-analysis, *International Archives of Allergy & Immunology*, **144**, 1–9.

Choonara, I. (2003). Safety of herbal medicines in children, *Archives of Disease in Childhood*, **88**, 1032–1033.

Daniels, J., Shaw, D., and Atherton, D. (2002). Use of wau wa in dermatitis patients, *Lancet*, **360**, 1025.

Dattner, A.M. (2003). From medical herbalism to phytotherapy in dermatology: Back to the future, *Dermatologic Therapy*, **16**, 106–13.

De Medeiros, L.M., Franway, A.F., Taylor, J.S., Wyman, M., Janes, J., Fowler, J.F., Jr., and Rietschel, R.L. (2008). Complementary and alternative remedies: An additional source of potential systemic nickel exposure, *Contact Dermatitis*, **58**, 97–100.

Ehlers, A., Stangier, U., and Gieler, U. (1995). Treatment of atopic dermatitis: A comparison of psychological and dermatological approaches to relapse prevention, *Journal of Consulting and Clinical Psychology*, **63**, 624–635.

Eisenberg, D.M., Davis, R.B., Ettner, S.L., Appel, S., Wilkey, S., Van Rompay, M., and Kessler, R.C. (1998). Trends in alternative medicine use in the united states, 1990–1997: Results of a follow-up national survey, *Journal of the American Medical Association*, **280**, 1569–1575.

Ernst, E. (2000). Adverse effects of herbal drugs in dermatology, *British Journal of Dermatology*, **143**, 923–929.

Ernst, E., Pittler, M.H., and Stevenson, C. (2002). Complementary/alternative Medicine in dermatology: Evidence-assessed efficacy of two diseases and two treatments, *American Journal of Clinical Dermatology*, **3**, 341–348.

Farag, R.S., Shalaby, A.S., El-Baroty, G.A., Ibrahim, N.A., Ali, M.A., and Hassan, E.M. (2004). Chemical and biological evaluation of the essential oils of different melaleuca species, *Phytotherapy Research*, **18**, 30–35.

Ferguson, J.E., Chalmers, R.J., and Rowlands, D.J. (1997). Reversible dilated cardiomyopathy following treatment of atopic eczema with chinese herbal medicine, *British Journal of Dermatology*, **136**, 592–593.

Fisher, P., Van Hasalen, R., Hardy, K., Berkovitz, S., and McCarney, R. (2004). Effectiveness gaps: A new concept for evaluating health service and research needs applied to complementary and alternative medicine, *Journal of Alternative & Complementary Medicine*, **10**, 627–632.

Fleischer, A.B., Jr., Feldman, S.R., Rapp, S.R., Reboussin, D.M., Exum, M.L., and Clark, A.R. (1996). Alternative therapies commonly used within a population of patients with psoriasis, *Cutis*, **58**, 216–220.

Fuhrmann, T., Smith, N., and Tausk, F. (2009). Use of complementary and alternative medicine among adults with skin disease: Updated results from a national survey, *Journal of the American Academy of Dermatology*, **63**, 1000–1005.

Fung, A.Y., Look, P.C., Chong, L.Y., But, P.P., and Wong, E. (1999). A controlled trial of traditional Chinese herbal medicine in Chinese patients with recalcitrant atopic dermatitis, *International Journal of Dermatology*, **38**, 387–392.

Gelfand, J.M., Crawford, G.H., Brod, B.A., and Szazpary, P.O. (2005). Adverse cutaneous reactions to guggulipid, *Journal of the American Academy of Dermatology*, **52**, 533–534.

Gonul, M., Gul, U., Cakmak, S.K., and Kilic, S. (2009). Unconventional medicine in dermatology outpatients in Turkey, *International Journal of Dermatology*, **48**, 639–644.

Graham-Brown, R. (2000). Atopic dermatitis: Unapproved treatments or indications, *Clinical Dermatology*, **18**, 153–158.

Henderson, C.A., Morris, A., Wilson, A., and Iiychshyn, A. (2000). An open study comparing the efficacy of two different Chinese herbal formulations in atopic eczema and their effects on circulating activated T-lymphocytes, *Journal of Dermatological Treatment*, **11(2)**, 91–96.

Hoare, C., Li Wan Po, A., and Williams, H. (2000). Systematic review of treatments for atopic eczema, *Health Technology Assessment*, **4**, 1–191.

Hon, K.L.E., Leung, T.F., and Ng, P.C. (2007). Efficacy and tolerability of a chinese herbal medicine concoction for treatment of atopic dermatitis: A randomized, double-blind, placebo-controlled study, *British Journal of Dermatology*, **157**, 357–363.

Hong, J., Koo, B., and Koo, J. (2008). The psychosocial and occupational impact of chronic skin disease, *Dermatologic Therapy*, **21**, 54–59.

Jellinek, N. and Maloney, M. E. (2005). Escharotic and other botanical agents for the treatment of skin cancer: A review, *Journal of the American Academy of Dermatology*, **53**, 487–495.

Jensen, P. (1990). Alternative therapy for atopic dermatitis and psoriasis: Patient-reported motivation, information source and effect, *Acta Dermato-Venereologica*, **70**, 425–428.

Johnston, G.A., Bilbao, R.M., and Graham-Brown, R.A. (2003). The use of complementary medicine in children with atopic dermatitis in secondary care in Leicester, *British Journal of Dermatology*, **149**, 566–571.

Kalliomaki, M., Salminen, S., Poussa, T., Arvilommi, H., and Isolauri, E. (2003). Probiotics and prevention of atopic disease: 4-year follow-up of a randomised placebo-controlled trial, *Lancet*, **361**, 1869–1871.

Keane, F.M., Munn, S.E., Du Vivier, A.W., Taylor, N.F., and Higgins, E.M. (1999). Analysis of Chinese herbal creams prescribed for dermatological conditions, *British Medical Journal*, **318**, 563–564.

Kessler, R.C., Davis, R.B., Foster, D.F., Van Rompay, M.I., Walters, E.E., Wilkey, S.A., Kaptchuk, T.J., and Eisenberg, D.M. (2001). Long-term trends in the use of complementary and alternative medical therapies in the United States, *Annals of Internal Medicine*, **135**, 262–268.

Kitai, E., Vinker, S., Sandiuk, A., Hornik, O., Zeltcer, C., and Gaver, A. (1998). Use of complementary and alternative medicine among primary care patients, *Family Practice*, **15**, 411–414.

Kitz, R., Rose, M.A., Schonborn, H., Zielen, S., and Bohles, H.J. (2006). Impact of early dietary gamma-linolenic acid supplementation on atopic eczema in infancy, *Pediatric Allergy & Immunology*, **17**, 112–127.

Koo, J. and Lebwohl, A. (2001). Psycho dermatology: the mind and skin connection, *American Family Physician*, **64**, 1873–1878.

Kuitunen, M., Kukkonen, K., Juntunen-Backman, K., Korpela, R., Poussa, T., Tuure, T., Haahtela, T., and Savilahti, E. (2009). Probiotics prevent ige-associated allergy until age 5 years in cesarean-delivered children but not in the total cohort, *Journal of Allergy and Clinical Immunology*, **123**, 335–341.

Kukkonen, K., Savilahti, E., Haahtela, T., Juntunen-Backman, K., Korpela, R., Poussa, T., Tuure, T., and Kuitunen, M. (2008). Long-term safety and impact on infection rates of postnatal probiotic and prebiotic (synbiotic) treatment: randomized, double-blind, placebo-controlled trial, *Pediatrics*, **122**, 8–12.

Lee, G.B.W., Charn, T.C., Chew, Z.H., Ng, T.P. (2004). Complementary and alternative medicine use in patients with chronic diseases in primary care is associated with perceived quality of care and cultural beliefs, *Family Practice* **21**, 654–660.

Lee, J. and Bielory, L. (2010). Complementary and alternative interventions in atopic dermatitis, *Immunology and Allergy Clinics of North America*, **30**, 411–424.

Linde, K., Jonas, W.B., Melchart, D., and Willich, S. (2001). The methodological quality of randomized controlled trials of homeopathy, herbal medicines and acupuncture, *International Journal of Epidemiology*, **30**, 526–531.

Lord, G.M., Cook, T., Arlt, V.M., Schmeiser, H.H., Williams, G., and Pusey, C.D. (2001). Urothelial malignant disease and chinese herbal nephropathy, *Lancet*, **358**, 1515–1516.

Lord, G.M., Tagore, R., Cook, T., Gower, P., and Pusey, C.D. (1999). Nephropathy caused by Chinese herbs in the UK, *Lancet*, **354**, 481–482.

Magin, P. and Adams, J. (2007). Complementary and alternative medicines: Use in skin diseases, *Expert Review of Dermatology*, **2**, 41–44.

Magin, P., Adams, J., Heading, G.S., and Pond, D. (2009). Patients with skin disease and their relationship with their doctors: Results of a qualitative study of acne, psoriasis and eczema, *Medical Journal of Australia*, **190**, 62–64.

Magin, P., Adams, J., Heading, G.S., Pond, D.C., and Smith, W. (2006a). Complementary and alternative medicine therapies in acne, psoriasis, and atopic eczema: Results of a qualitative study of patients' experiences and perceptions, *Journal of Alternative & Complementary Medicine*, **12**, 451–457.

Magin, P., Adams, J., Pond, C.D., and Smith, W. (2006b). Topical and oral CAM in acne: A review of the empirical evidence and a consideration of its context, *Complementary Therapies in Medicine*, **14**, 62–76.

Monk, B. (1986). Severe cutaneous reactions to alternative remedies, *British Medical Journal*, **293**, 665–666.

Morris, M.C., Donoghue, A., Markowitz, J.A., and Osterhoudt, K. C. (2003). Ingestion of tea tree oil (melaleuca oil) by a 4-year-old boy, *Pediatric Emergency Care*, **19**, 169–171.

Morse, P.F., Horrobin, D.F., Manku, M.S., Stewart, J.C., Allen, R., Littlewood, S., Wright, S., Burton, J., Gould, D.J., and Holt, P.J. (1989). Meta-analysis of placebo-controlled studies of the efficacy of epogam in the treatment of atopic eczema. Relationship between plasma essential fatty acid changes and clinical response, *British Journal of Dermatology*, **121**, 75–90.

Nicolaou, N. and Johnston, G.A. (2004). The use of complementary medicine by patients referred to a contact dermatitis clinic, *Contact Dermatitis*, **51**, 30–33.

Oguamanam, C. (2006). Biomedical orthodoxy and complementary and alternative medicine: ethical challenges of integrating medical cultures, *Journal of Alternative and Complementary Medicine*, **12**, 577–581.

Pieroni, A., Quave, C.L., Villanelli, M.L., Mangino, P., Sabbatini, G., Santini, L., Boccetti, T., Profili, M., Ciccioli, T., Rampa, L.G., Antonini, G., Girolamini, C., Cecchi, M., and Tomasi, M. (2004). Ethnopharmacognostic survey on the natural ingredients used in folk cosmetics, cosmeceuticals and remedies for healing skin diseases in the inland marches, central-eastern Italy, *Journal of Ethnopharmacology*, **91**, 331–344.

Pittler, M.H., Armstrong, N.C., Cox, A., Collier, P.M., Hart, A., and Ernst, E. (2003). Randomized, double-blind, placebo-controlled trial of autologous blood therapy for atopic dermatitis, *British Journal of Dermatology*, **148**, 307–313.

Ramsay, H.M., Goddard, W., Gill, S., and Moss, C. (2003). Herbal creams used for atopic eczema in Birmingham, UK illegally contain potent corticosteroids, *Archives of Disease in Childhood*, **88**, 1056–1057.

Schachner, L., Field, T., Hernandez-Reif, M., Duarte, A.M., and Krasnegor, J. (1998). Atopic dermatitis symptoms decreased in children following massage therapy, *Pediatric Dermatology*, **15**, 390–395.

See, A., Teo, B., Kwan, R., Lim, R., Lee, J., Tang, M.B.Y., and Verkooijen, H.M. (2011). Use of complementary and alternative medicine among dermatology outpatients in Singapore, *Australasian Journal of Dermatology*, **52**, 7–13.

Shapira, M.Y., Raphaelovich, Y., Gilad, L., Or, R., Dumb, A.J., and Ingber, A. (2005). Treatment of atopic dermatitis with herbal combination of eleutherococcus, achillea millefolium, and lamium album has no advantage over placebo: A double blind, placebo-controlled, randomized trial, *Journal of the American Academy of Dermatology*, **52**, 691–693.

Sharples, F.M., Van Haselen, R., and Fisher, P. (2003). NHS patients' perspective on complementary medicine: A survey, *Complementary Therapies in Medicine*, **11**, 243–248.

Sheehan, M.P. and Atherton, D.J. (1994). One-year follow up of children treated with chinese medicinal herbs for atopic eczema, *British Journal of Dermatology*, **130**, 488–493.

Sheehan, M.P., Rustin, M.H., Atherton, D.J., Buckley, C., Harris, D.W., Brostoff, J., Ostlere, L., and Dawson, A. (1992). Efficacy of traditional chinese herbal therapy in adult atopic dermatitis, *Lancet*, **340**, 13–17.

Sheehan, M.P., Stevens, H., Ostlere, L.S., Atherton, D.J., Brostoff, J., and Rustin, M.H. (1995). Follow-up of adult patients with atopic eczema treated with Chinese herbal therapy for 1 year, *Clinical and Experimental Dermatology*, **20**, 136–140.

Smith, N., Shin, D.B., Brauer, J.A., Mao J., and Gelfand, J.M. (2009). Use of complementary and alternative medicine among adults with skin disease: Results from a national survey, *Journal of the American Academy of Dermatology*, **60**, 419–425.

Sollner, W., Zingg-Schir, M., Rumpold, G., and Fritsch, P. (1997). Attitude toward alternative therapy, compliance with standard treatment, and need for emotional support in patients with melanoma, *Archives of Dermatology*, **133**, 316–321.

Stewart, A.C. and Thomas, S.E. (1995). Hypnotherapy as a treatment for atopic dermatitis in adults and children, *British Journal of Dermatology*, **132**, 778–783.

Thorne, S., Best, A., Balon, J., Kelner, M., and Rickhi, B. (2002). Ethical dimensions in the borderland between conventional and complementary/alternative medicine, *Journal of Alternative and Complementary Medicine*, **8**, 907–915.

Uehara, M., Sugiura, H., and Sakurai, K. (2001). A trial of oolong tea in the management of recalcitrant atopic dermatitis, *Archives of Dermatology*, **137**, 42–43.

Van Gool, C.J., Zeegers, M.P., and Thijs, C. (2004). Oral essential fatty acid supplementation in atopic dermatitis: A meta-analysis of placebo-controlled trials, *British Journal of Dermatology*, **150**, 728–740.

Ventura, M.T., Viola, M., Calogiuri, G., Gaeta, F., Pesole, O., and Romano, A. (2006). Hypersensitivity reactions to complementary and alternative medicine products, *Current Pharmaceutical Design*, **12**, 3393–3399.

Verucchi, G., Calza, L., Attard, L., and Chiodo, F. (2002). Acute hepatitis induced by traditional Chinese herbs used in the treatment of psoriasis, *Journal of Gastroenterology and Hepatology*, **17**, 1342–1343.

Vohra, S. and Cohen, M.H. (2007). Ethics of complementary and alternative medicine use in children, *Pediatric Clinics of North America*, **54**, 875–884.

Williams, A.M., Kitchen, P., and Eby, J. (2011). Alternative health care consultations in Ontario, Canada: A geographic and socio-demographic analysis, *BMC Complementary and Alternative Medicine*, **11**, 47.

Yarnell, E. and Abascal, K. (2006). Herbal medicine for acne vulgaris, *Alternative and Complementary Therapies*, **12**, 303–309.

Zhang, W., Leonard, T., Bath-Hextall, F., Chambers, C.A., Lee, C., Humphreys, R., and Williams, H.C. (2004). Chinese herbal medicine for atopic eczema, *Cochrane Database of Systematic Reviews*, **4**, CD002291.

Part Two

Practitioners and the Professional CIM Interface

CHAPTER 4

Naturopaths: Their Role in Primary Health Care Delivery

Jon Wardle and Jon Adams

4.1 Challenges in Primary Health Care

Complementary and integrative medicine (CIM) is playing an increasingly important role in the delivery of health care — including primary health care (PHC) — in countries around the world. Naturopaths in particular are becoming major providers of CIM services in Southern African, South Asian, Australasian, European, Middle Eastern, and North American countries. This chapter will explore the potential role that naturopaths may play in PHC, where appropriate, and discuss relevant practice, regulatory, and legislative developments that should be part of any naturopathic role in PHC delivery.

The development of a strong PHC infrastructure is associated not only with delivering better health care outcomes and lower costs of health care delivery, but also delivering a more equitable health care system (Starfield *et al.*, 2005). Comparisons at local, state, and international levels have consistently shown that having a greater percentage of the physician workforce engaged in PHC specialties is associated with better population health outcomes, including significant improvements in all-cause, cardiovascular, cancer-specific, and infant mortality (Macinko *et al.*, 2007).

Compounding issues include the recruitment and retention of conventional PHC providers in underserved areas and the decreasing number of conventional providers choosing to enter PHC more generally (Bodenheimer, 2006). Therefore, medical pluralism, or the extension of other health care providers into PHC has been seen as one way of alleviating PHC provider shortages. For example, in the United States conventional PHC is served by medical doctors (MDs) and osteopathic doctors (DOs), and the historic decline in MD numbers since the 1950s had been historically ameliorated by the high numbers of DOs that pursued a career in PHC.

This was thought to be due largely to the nurturing of PHC education in osteopathic schools and colleges (Cummings *et al.*, 2006). However, there is now debate as to whether the traditionally high proportion of DOs entering PHC has been related more to training philosophy or to reduced access to specialist residencies (Cummings and Dobbs, 2005), an argument that gains strength considering the fact that the proportion of DOs now entering PHC is following the same downward trend as MDs access to specialist residencies (Robert Graham Center, 2005).

As conventional practitioner PHC numbers have declined, new types of providers have been considered. Emerging professions such as nurse practitioners and physician assistants are being increasingly used to fill gaps in primary care delivery (Naylor and Kurtzman, 2010). Although often controversial, the incorporation of non-medical practitioner PHC providers has generally been successful in improving access to primary care services, with little evidence of patient care being compromised, and some elements even being improved (Horrocks *et al.*, 2002).

Given the success of incorporating new professions into PHC delivery, it is worthwhile considering what other professions may house potential for providing PHC services in areas of unmet need. This may include extending consideration to CIM providers. One CIM profession that may warrant exploration as a potential option for improving access to PHC is naturopathic medicine, or naturopathy.

4.2 Naturopathy

Naturopathy is a distinct system of PHC medicine that blends Western healing traditions with modern medical theory. The profession defines itself as a system of primary health care: an art, science and philosophy, and practice of diagnosis, treatment, and prevention of illness. Like other "systems" of medicine, such as Ayurvedic and Chinese medicine, naturopathy is not defined by individual tools of practice (such as homoeopathy or acupuncture) but by the principles and philosophies by which these tools are used. The central principles that underlie and determine the practice of naturopathy include: supporting the healing power of nature (the *Vis medicatrix naturae*); determining and treating the underlying cause of health imbalances, rather than focusing on symptomatic treatment; treating the whole person, rather than individual disease processes; prevention of disease and perceiving the practitioner as a teacher (Sarris and Wardle, 2010).

Also central to naturopathic philosophy is the concept of a therapeutic order of interventions, which places emphasis on prevention and less forceful interventions before resorting to more interventionist healing strategies (Zeff *et al.*, 2008). This therapeutic order consists of: (i) establishing the conditions of health by identifying and removing factors and instituting a health regimen, (ii) stimulating self-healing mechanisms or the *Vis medicatrix naturae*; (iii) supporting weakened or damaged organs or systems, (iv) addressing the pathology using specific natural substances, modalities or interventions, (v) addressing the pathology using specific synthetic or pharmacological interventions, and (vi) suppressing or surgically removing pathology. This principle gives naturopaths a flexible and broad scope of interventions, and allows them to work and integrate well with other medical systems.

Although not limited to the use of "natural" therapies — in fact North American naturopaths enjoy broad prescriptive authority in several jurisdictions (Baer and Sporn, 2009) — the major modalities utilized by naturopathic medicine practitioners tend to fall within the "natural" medicine remit (Boon *et al.*, 2004). These include dietary and clinical nutritional interventions, herbal medicine, homoeopathy, hydrotherapy, physical medicine, lifestyle and behavioural interventions, physical medicine, traditional nature cure, and tools incorporated from other traditions (such as acupuncture). The focus of naturopaths on the underlying philosophies and principles of their discipline has allowed the profession to develop a broad therapeutic eclecticism, and for this reason naturopaths often perceive themselves as analogous to general practitioners of complementary and alternative medicine (CAM) (Wardle *et al.*, 2010).

It should be noted, however, that this eclecticism has also resulted in significant differences in naturopathic medicine communities internationally.

In India, naturopathy was popularized by Gandhi, who was influenced by the original nature cure teachings of Kniepp, Kuhne, Just, and Lindlahr, and has largely retained this focus on nature cure and the avoidance of ingestible medicines as well as incorporating yoga practices (Alter, 2004). In Britain, the shared history of naturopathic medicine and osteopathic medicine has meant that a greater focus on physical medicine and osteopathic manipulation are seen in naturopathy in that country (Chaitow, 2008). In North America, continental Europe, Africa, and Australasia, naturopathic practitioners utilize a broad scope of natural therapies, with a greater focus on ingestive and interventionist therapies (Baer and Sporn, 2009).

However, even within countries variability can exist. The unregulated nature of the profession in Australia has led to an extraordinary variability of practitioners, with many practitioners having no naturopathic qualification or training at all (Lin *et al.*, 2005). In North America, similar variability is observed across licensed and unlicensed naturopaths: although in licensed states naturopaths are required to have completed a four-year postgraduate curriculum with similar medical science training to conventional medical providers, in unlicensed states naturopaths may operate without any training at all (Hough *et al.*, 2001).

4.3 The Naturopathic Practice of Primary Health Care

Although the incorporation of naturopathic medicine into broader PHC may pose several challenges, there may be certain situations where naturopaths provide improvements over existing PHC services. The significant problems with recruitment and retention of PHC providers in underserved areas (such as rural areas) (Tolhurst *et al.*, 2006) may make integrating naturopaths or other non-conventional providers into PHC a more palatable option, particularly where no other care options exist. Significant numbers of naturopaths may already exist in areas of health provider shortage and represent a potential untapped resource for PHC delivery. For example, an audit of CIM providers in rural New South Wales, Australia, found that the number of "PHC" CAM providers (naturopathy, Chinese medicine, chiropractic, homeopathy, and osteopathy) was nearly as high as the number of conventional GPs in those areas (Wardle *et al.*, 2011).

Several precedents exist for the use of naturopathic practitioners in underserved areas. For example, in Germany naturopaths (*Heilpraktiker*) are able to perform publicly subsidized PHC services in rural areas if conventional PHC services are not available (Bodeker and Burford, 2007). In the United States, accredited naturopaths practising or willing to practise in areas of need or underserved communities are eligible for state loan forgiveness programmes in Washington and Oregon or the federal scheme for service in the US *Indian Health Service* (United States Department of Health and Human Services, 2012).

4.4 Conventional Provider Perceptions of Primary Health Care and Alignment with Naturopathic Practice and Philosophy

Conventional PHC providers often see themselves as different to other doctors (Adams, 2001a, 2001b; Tovey and Adams, 2001). Beyond the clinical treatment of patients, PHC providers may also act as patient advocates in both the self-management and co-management of care, acting as the patient's representative in — and helping to guide them through — an increasingly complex and multifaceted health system (Stange, 2010). Such a role requires skill sets that extend beyond the clinical realm into the psychosocial model. Naturopaths, who like many other CIM therapists have an underlying holistic and patient-centred philosophy, may have already developed the skills required to take on this aspect of PHC.

Additionally, the clinical skills required to practise in a PHC capacity are unique in medicine. The reasons for visits to PHC practitioners are incredibly diverse, with only one half of reasons for visits classified in the top 20 diagnosis clusters (Schneeweiss *et al.*, 1986; Stange *et al.*, 1998). This compares with the top six diagnostic clusters forming 70–90% of patient presentations in specialties such as cardiology or dermatology (Schneeweiss *et al.*, 1986). This heterogeneity highlights the importance of a PHC specialist developing a broad, general knowledge of medicine, coupled with developing a utilizable resource network when deeper expertise is required. In many respects, only a generalist can be a true "PHC practitioner", as specializing automatically limits the scope of practice from a largely co-management or consultative role to a narrower range of presentations.

A generalist approach to health care employed in PHC involves work-ing on the parts while paying attention to the whole (Stange, 2002). Stange (2009) posits that whilst specialist and narrowly focused approaches are clinically useful, the generalist approach is most important in complex situations in PHC, such as times of transition and instability, circum-stances involving ambiguity and variability, situations where relationships and individualization matter, systems with a high degree of interconnect-edness or complexity, settings in which both strongly and loosely related events unfold with time, and situations where the whole is more than the sum of its parts. This approach has clear parallels with the holistic and patient-centred approach associated with CIM practice observed in natur-opathic medicine — one that often attracts PHC physicians themselves to CIM (Adams, 2001a; Adams, 2001b; Adams, 2003).

4.5 Naturopaths and Responsive Care

Engaging naturopaths into PHC delivery may also be an appropriate response to the changing demands of health care users, who are actively seeking the services of CIM providers. An estimated 69% of Australians used CIM in 2005, spending approximately USD 3.1 billion out-of-pocket (Xue *et al.*, 2007). The estimated 40% of Americans who use CIM spend nearly USD 34 billion out-of-pocket (Barnes *et al.*, 2008). The majority of complementary medicine users in the US (58%) appear to use CIM for *prevention* of disease, as opposed to *treating* disease (42%) (Barnes *et al.*, 2008). This also aligns with the self-identified principles of PHC practice of naturopathic practitioners, who suggest that the naturopathic model of PHC focuses on prevention rather than reactive treatment (Wardle *et al.*, 2010).

Naturopaths are often already providing PHC services for many patients, albeit frequently in an unofficial or undocumented capacity, and incorporation may allow better documentation and accountability of naturopathic PHC practice. In Australia, despite universal health coverage for conventional services and little integration of naturopathy into the broader health sector, 11% of mid-age women still choose to consult (and pay out-of-pocket) a naturopath (Adams *et al.*, 2007). This use often rises in complex or chronic conditions, for example, in cancer this can increase to 16% (Adams *et al.*, 2005). Significant use of naturopaths in serious conditions such as cancer is itself a potent argument for further incorporation of naturopaths into conventional health systems — at least in terms of ensuring accountability and minimum practice standards.

Although most naturopathic patients seek the services of CAM practitioners in an adjunctive capacity with other health practitioners, there is a significant portion that utilize them as their primary point-of-care or first contact practitioners. In Australia, for example, it has been estimated that one third of Australian naturopathic patients use their naturopaths as their PHC providers (Chow, 2000; Grace *et al.*, 2006). Incorporating naturopaths into health service delivery may also assist in developing more responsive conventional medical care, as exploring and documenting the reasons behind naturopathic practitioner use in PHC can identify the gaps that naturopaths are filling, and develop responsive PHC services to address these needs.

4.6 A Role for Naturopathic Medicine Due to Changing Primary Health Care Priorities

The public health shift to focusing on non-communicable diseases may uncover opportunities to utilize naturopaths in PHC. Chronic diseases are now the leading cause of disease burden and morbidity internationally, yet the leading underlying actual causes of death are all modifiable health behaviours: tobacco use, poor diet and physical inactivity (Nugent, 2008). The principles of naturopathy may align well with efforts to face these challenges, and the potential of the intersecting paradigms of naturopathic medicine and public health have been discussed previously (Adams, 2008; Wardle and Oberg, 2011).

For example, health promotion is a cornerstone of naturopathy, both philosophically and in care delivery (Herman *et al.*, 2006; Nahin *et al.*, 2007). Naturopaths facilitate individual behavioural change in patients both through the clinical delivery of health promotion counselling and also by modelling healthy behaviours themselves (Frank *et al.*, 2000). Observational studies of naturopathic practice indicate that health promotion counselling on diet, physical activity and stress management is incorporated into almost every clinical encounter (80–100%) and is then reinforced over successive patient visits (Bradley and Oberg 2006; Bradley *et al.*, 2009). This contrasts with the lower rates of health promotion activity observed in conventional care, which range between 35% and 40% (Ma *et al.*, 2004).

Additionally, naturopaths are being increasingly sought by patients with chronic or complex conditions. A review of the PHC practice patterns of 170 naturopaths in Washington and Connecticut suggests that 75% of all patient visits to naturopaths were for chronic conditions (Boon *et al.*, 2004). Naturopaths also self-identify their greatest strengths in the areas of chronic and complex disease: a qualitative exploration conducted in rural Australia also shows that naturopaths claim to provide more responsive PHC to chronic patients than conventional providers, whereas conventional providers were perceived by these same naturopaths as better at providing acute care (Wardle *et al.*, 2010).

4.7 Challenges Incorporating Naturopaths into Primary Care

4.7.1 *Distribution of naturopathic practitioners*

Although the number of naturopaths in North America is increasing, with a 91% increase in the five years between 2001 and 2006 (Albert and Martinez, 2006), the current distribution of naturopaths may not be immediately amenable to increasing their role in delivering essential PHC services. For example, the distribution of naturopaths in the United States is largely predicted by population density and distance from naturopathic medical school (Albert and Butar, 2004). This seems to suggest that the current distribution of naturopaths serves only to complement existing access to health services, rather than increasing access to PHC services across the broader population.

However, examination of naturopathic practitioner distribution in the US has suggested that naturopaths could play a role in reducing health provider shortages. It has been estimated that the number of designated US counties with official federal designation as a single county PHC Health Professional Shortage Area could be reduced by up to 142 if naturopathic doctors (NDs) were included in PHC professionals (Albert and Butar, 2005). What remains clear is that if naturopaths are to have a greater role in PHC delivery, more naturopaths need to be operating in areas that are not already well-served by conventional providers.

Such refocusing may increase the PHC capacity of naturopaths. For example, Australian naturopaths practising in rural areas found that their capacity to perform PHC was increased in rural practice as opposed to urban practice, and that this was due not only to the health workforce shortage of conventional health care providers, but to the cultural affinity of rural Australia to naturopathic services (Wardle *et al.*, 2010).

4.7.2 *Risks of naturopathic practice*

The practice of naturopathic medicine carries with it substantial enough risk to make statutory regulation of practitioners both desirable and warranted (Lin *et al.*, 2005). Although the therapies utilized by naturopathic practitioners do carry some direct health risks, for example, naturopathic treatments negatively interacting with conventional treatment, it is the indirect and non-health risks of naturopathic treatment which pose the most risk to the consumer (Wardle and Adams, 2012). These may include missed diagnoses (or misdiagnoses), failure to refer patients when clinically appropriate, or the inappropriate monopolization of PHC. However, reviews of the naturopathic profession have indicated that these risks can be significantly decreased through regulation of the profession that places suitable barriers to entry for people practising — most importantly via minimum education standards and character tests (Lin *et al.*, 2005).

One of the major risks to public safety associated with an increased role for naturopaths in PHC delivery is the potential for conflicts of interest to result in financial exploitation of patients, due to the fact that prescription and sale of therapeutic interventions are not typically separated in naturopathic practice. For example, 98% of Australian naturopaths have a dispensary for extemporaneous medicines in their clinic, and 78% sell pre-packaged products directly to their patients (Smith *et al.*, 2005). This is often not simply a commercial decision by practitioners, but is also considered necessary for the preparation of individualized medicines or in the absence of third-party suppliers of naturopathic medicines, and was possibly a solution derived due to the long-term isolation of the naturopathic profession from conventional health infrastructure. These risks can also be ameliorated not just through the development of third-party dispensing options, but also through the development of appropriate regulatory policies (Parker *et al.*, 2011).

4.7.3 *Fringe therapies and practitioner variability*

A common criticism of naturopaths — and a common argument often used against their regulation before assessment on risk-based criteria became the norm — is the illegitimate nature of many of their therapies. When passing down its recommendation not to regulate naturopathy in 1977, the taskforce employed by the Australian Government to explore naturopathic regulation suggested that naturopathy was a "minor cult system" and that it should not be registered as it "may give a form of official imprimatur to practices which the Committee considers unscientific and, at best, of marginal efficacy" (Webb, 1977, p. 99).

However, such marginalization can be counter-productive and ultimately self-fulfilling. Gort and Coburn (1988) describe how naturopathic medicine in Canada was in many ways increasingly defined by its marginal status, which resulted in the profession absorbing increasingly marginal "alternative" therapies and taking oppositional stances that were irrelevant to its underlying principles or philosophies, as it rebelled against the mainstream medical hegemony. The promotion of fringe therapies is also exacerbated by the variability of naturopathic training in unregulated jurisdictions. For example, a survey of the Australian naturopathic workforce showed that 10% of naturopaths practising in that country had no formal naturopathic training at all, and a significant number of practitioners had only minor vocational qualifications in other complementary therapies (Bensoussan *et al.*, 2004).

Whorton (2004) also suggests that the naïveté of the naturopathic profession in North America may have led it to absorb, and ultimately be dominated by, fringe or alternative movements in the 1960s and 1970s that were largely unrelated to its underpinning philosophy. Baer (2006) posits that this co-option of naturopathic medicine by "alternative" medicine in Australia occurred as the "new style flower children began to join the 'old style straight-backed nature cure adherents'". Whereas older naturopathic practitioners embraced the scientific process and saw it as a tool with which to validate and promote their therapeutic practices, these new practitioners were largely suspicious of the scientific movement, and often were attracted to naturopathic medicine as an act of rebellion against the scientific movement (Whorton, 2004).

However, improved regulatory environments and the decreasingly marginalized nature of naturopathy appear to have reduced fringe therapies in the profession, which has restored focus on its underlying principles. More importantly, as education standards increase due to regulation enforcing minimum standards of health science and medical training, naturopathic practitioners are increasingly integrating with conventional health care services, rather than opposing them (Sarris and Wardle, 2010).

Institutional support for the inclusion of naturopaths without regulating minimum standards may not be appropriate, and may in fact lead to gains that have been made over the past few decades being lost. For example, the historically high levels of government funding for naturopathic education in Australia coupled with the recent failed attempt to statutorily regulate naturopaths in the state of Victoria have resulted not just in a decline of naturopathic education standards, but a decline in research and other academic activity in that profession as well (Wardle *et al.*, 2012a).

4.7.4 *The relevance of naturopathic medicine to broad populations*

It also remains to be seen whether naturopaths are able to provide PHC services to broad populations. International studies routinely demonstrate that the typical naturopathic patient is generally wealthier, "whiter" and better educated than the average population (Adams *et al.*, 2003; Conboy *et al.*, 2005; Adams *et al.*, 2007; Barnes *et al.*, 2008; Steinsbekk *et al.*, 2009). However, those who could potentially benefit the most from an extension of new providers into PHC often fall outside of this demographic. The only disadvantaged group that appear to be currently served by naturopathic medicine are rural patients, with some studies suggesting that use of naturopathic practitioners is higher amongst non-urban residents than for urban residents (Wardle *et al.*, 2012b). This may be due to the unsubsidized nature of many naturopathic treatments, or the lack of integration of naturopaths into conventional health care delivery.

Although the underlying principles of naturopathy would seem to suggest it possesses the flexibility to serve diverse patient populations, active efforts need to be undertaken by the profession to demonstrate that naturopathic medicine can achieve the same PHC outcomes in vulnerable and disadvantaged populations as achieved in patients of higher socio-economic status.

4.7.5 *Length of consultation*

Given the increased length of naturopathic consultation times, which average 40 minutes, when compared with conventional providers, incorporating naturopathic practitioners may not necessarily equate to high levels of full-time practice and provision (Boon *et al.*, 2003). However, naturopaths themselves perceive that the therapeutic relationship engendered by longer consultation times is an advantage in PHC, suggesting that it can improve patient compliance with treatment and ultimately reduce the need for follow-up visits and be seen as "better value for money" by patients (Wardle *et al.*, 2010).

Although longer consultation times may help present the immediate potential PHC footprint of naturopaths as less than conventional providers, this disadvantage may be neutralized by longer term benefits. An evaluation of complementary medicine practices in Germany found that despite an increase in consultation times, minor cost savings (4.2%) were achieved and the patients exhibited long-term stable reduction of chronic disease (a 46% reduction in disease scores and a 43% reduction in symptom scores) and a 14% increase in health related quality-of-life scores (Hamre *et al.*, 2004).

4.8 Regulation of Naturopaths

Some jurisdictions have long-standing regulation of naturopathic practitioners. In the United States naturopaths have been licensed since 1919 (Washington State) and in Canada (Ontario) since 1925 (Whorton, 2004). Yet, many US states and Canadian provinces remain unregulated.

Naturopaths remain completely unregulated in Australia — where naturopathic history has been equally as long and the popular utilization of naturopaths as health providers arguably more entrenched. The regulation of naturopaths in Australia has been a matter of political discussion since 1925, when the first formal debates on the issue were made in the South Australian parliament (Clark-Nikola, 1925), and the first government recommendation for regulation of the profession occurred in 1975 (Victorian Parliament Joint Select Committee, 1975). The legislative environment in Europe is varied, with naturopaths remaining unregulated in the United Kingdom but being licensed by some jurisdictions in Germany and Switzerland. Several African and Asian nations also regulate naturopathic medicine practitioners (Bodeker and Burford, 2007). The continuing rise in consumer demand and increasing numbers of naturopathic medical graduates practising PHC medicine provide the legislative impetus to define and regulate the practice of naturopathic practitioners (White House Commission on Complementary and Alternative Medicine Policy, 2002; Lin *et al.*, 2005; Verhoef *et al.*, 2006). Any role that naturopaths can play in PHC is dependent on the appropriate regulatory and legislative safeguards.

4.9 The Legislative Environment for Naturopaths in PHC Practice

Naturopaths are licensed as PHC providers in 15 US states and territories (Fleming and Gutknecht, 2010). Recent health reforms in the United States, enabled through the passing of the *Patient Protection and Affordable Health Care Act (HR 3590)*, have introduced new opportunities for implementing these licensed naturopaths in PHC delivery. The non-discrimination clause (Section 2706 of the Act) requires that third-party payers "shall not discriminate with respect to participation under the plan or coverage against any health care provider who is acting within the scope of that provider's license or certification under applicable State law". Given the broad scope of practice US NDs enjoy in states with naturopathic licensure, this alone would significantly increase the role NDs may play in PHC, as non-discrimination clauses were not previously enacted in the few states with naturopathic licensure.

Naturopaths are also included in sections of the Act related to health care payment, delivery, research and workforce: the Act requires that complementary and integrative medicine practitioners recognized by state licensure be included in the development of medical homes and community health teams (Section 3502); that they be adequately represented on the National Prevention, Health Promotion and Public Health Council (Section 4001); that they be included in national health workforce strategy (Section 5101) and that they also be included in the development of a patient-centred research initiative (Section 6301).

The role that Canadian naturopaths may play in PHC is still being determined, particularly with major new regulatory changes such as the province of Ontario's *Naturopathy Act 2007*, which are still in the transitional phase. In common law countries such as Australia and the United Kingdom, unregistered naturopaths are allowed to provide health care services without significant barriers, beyond the use of restricted medicines or acts (limited to dental acts, prescription of optical devices and cervical spine manipulation in Australia). However, their unregulated nature leaves them largely excluded from public PHC delivery and they operate largely in the private sector in these countries.

4.10 Models for Incorporation

For the North American jurisdictions where amenable legislation exists, naturopaths may be able to assume a direct role in PHC, one that fully integrates into conventional health systems (such as medical homes). In other jurisdictions, naturopaths may be better utilized as part of a multidisciplinary health care team, as practice restrictions or deficiencies in training may prevent them from taking a more active leadership role in PHC.

4.11 Conclusion

Given the challenges facing attempts to ensure equitable access to PHC services it is possible to consider naturopaths as a potential untapped resource. However, despite the advantages the further incorporation of naturopaths into PHC brings, it also presents challenges associated with practitioner variability and patient risk. With the development of appropriate regulatory and quality policies, this health care resource may attract careful attention amongst other options with regards to future PHC policy and service planning in countries in which naturopaths have a major presence. Additionally, the significant presence and high prevalence of use of naturopaths — many of whom are already providing informal PHC services — should itself also serve as an impetus to reform naturopathic service delivery and regulatory policy.

References

Adams, J. (2001a). Enhancing holism? GPs' explanations of their complementary practice, *Complementary Health Practice Review*, **6(3)**, 193–204.

Adams, J. (2001b). Direct integrative practice, time constraints and reactive strategy: An examination of general practitioner therapists' perceptions of their complementary medicine, *Journal of Management in Medicine*, **15(4)**, 312–322.

Adams, J. (2003). The positive gains of integration: a qualitative study of general practitioner therapists' views of their complementary practice, *Primary Health Care Research and Development*, **4(2)**, 158–167.

Adams, J. (2008). Utilising and promoting the public health and health services research of complementary and alternative medicine: The founding of NORPHCAM, *Complementary Therapies in Medicine*, **16**, 24–25.

Adams, J., Sibbritt, D., Easthope, G., and Young, A. (2003). The profile of women who consult alternative health practitioners in Australia, *Medical Journal of Australia*, **179(6)**, 297–300.

Adams, J., Sibbritt, D., and Young, A. (2005). Naturopathy/herbalism consultations by mid-aged Australian women who have cancer, *European Journal of Cancer Care,* **14(5)**, 443–447.

Adams, J., Sibbritt, D., and Young, A. (2007). Consultations with a naturopath or herbalist: The prevalence of use and profile of users amongst mid-aged women in Australia, *Public Health*, **121(12)**, 954–957.

Albert, D. and Butar, F. (2004). Distribution, concentration, and health care implications of naturopathic physicians in the United States, *Complementary Health Practice Review*, **9(2)**, 103–117.

Albert, D. and Butar, F. (2005). Estimating the de-designation of single-county HPSAs in the United States by counting naturopathic physicians as medical doctors, *Applied Geography,* **25(3)**, 271–285.

Albert, D. and Martinez, D. (2006). The supply of naturopathic physicians in the United States and Canada continues to increase, *Complementary Health Practice Review,* **11(2)**, 120–122.

Alter, J. (2004). *Yoga in Modern India: The Body Between Philosophy and Science,* Princeton University Press, Princeton.

Baer, H. (2006). The drive for legitimation in Australian naturopathy: Successes and dilemmas, *Social Science and Medicine,* **63(7)**, 1771–1783.

Baer, H. and Sporn, S. (2009). *Naturopathy Around the World: Variations and Political Dilemmas of an Eclectic Heterdox Medical System,* Nova Science Publishers, New York.

Barnes, P., Bloom, B., and Nahin, R. (2008). *Complementary and Alternative Medicine Use Among Adults and Children: United States, 2007,* Hyattsville, U.S. Department of Health and Human Services, Division of Health Interview Statistics, Centers for Disease Control and Prevention, National Center for Health Statistics.

Bensoussan, A., Myers, S., Wu, S., and O'Connor, K. (2004). Naturopathic and Western herbal medicine practice in Australia: A workforce survey, *Complementary Therapies in Medicine,* **12(1)**, 17–27.

Bodeker, G. and Burford, G. (2007). *Traditional, Complementary and Alternative Medicine: Policy and Public Health Perspectives,* Imperial College Press, London.

Bodenheimer, T. (2006). Primary care: Will it survive? *New England Journal of Medicine,* **355(9)**, 861–864.

Boon, H., Cherkin, D., Erro, J., Sherman, K., Milliman, B., Booker, J., Cramer, E., Smith, E., Deyo, R., and Eisenberg, D. (2004). Practice patterns of naturopathic physicians: Eesults from a random survey of licensed practitioners in two US States, *BMC Complementary and Alternative Medicine,* **4**, 14.

Boon, H., Stewart, M., Kennard, M., and Guimond, J. (2003). Visiting family physicians and naturopathic practitioners. Comparing patient-practitioner interactions, *Canadian Family Physician,* **49**, 1481–1487.

Bradley, R. and Oberg, E.B. (2006). Naturopathic medicine and type 2 diabetes: A retrospective analysis from an academic clinic, *Alternative Medicine Reviews,* **11(1)**, 30–39.

Bradley, R., Kozura, E., Buckle, H., Kaltunas, J., Taish, S., and Standish, L. (2009). Description of clinical risk factor changes during naturopathic care for type 2 diabetes, *Journal of Alternative and Complementary Medicine*, **15(6)**, 633–638.

Chaitow, L. (ed.) (2008). *Naturopathic Physical Medicine: Theory and Practice for Manual Therapists and Naturopaths*, Churchill Livingstone, Edinburgh.

Chow, R. (2000). Complementary medicine: Impact on medical practice, *Current Therapeutics*, **41**, 76–79.

Clark-Nikola, H. (1925). Non-conformist medical practitioners: Should they be legally registered? *Nature Cure and Medical Freedom*, **1(3)**, 6–7.

Conboy, L., Patel, S., Kaptchuk, T., Gottlieb, B., Eisenberg, D., and Acevedo-Garcia, D. (2005). Sociodemographic determinants of the utilization of specific types of complementary and alternative medicine: An analysis based on a nationally representative survey sample, *Journal of Alternative and Complementary Medicine*, **11(6)**, 977–994.

Cummings, M. and Dobbs, K. (2005). The irony of osteopathic medicine and primary care, *Academic Medicine*, **80(7)**, 702–705.

Cummings, M., Kunkle, J., and Doane, C. (2006). Family medicine's search for manpower: The American Osteopathic Association accreditation option, *Family Medicine*, **38(3)**, 206–210.

Fleming, S. and Gutknecht, N. (2010). Naturopathy and the primary care practice, *Primary Care*, **37(1)**, 119–136.

Frank, E., Breyan, J., and Elon, L. (2000). Physician disclosure of healthy personal behaviors improves credibility and ability to motivate, *Archives of Family Medicine*, **9(3)**, 287–290.

Gort, E. and Coburn, D. (1988). Naturopathy in Canada: Changing relationships to medicine, chiropractic and the state, *Social Science and Medicine*, **26(10)**, 1061–1072.

Grace, S., Vemulpad, S., and Beirman, R. (2006). Training in and use of diagnostic techniques among CAM practitioners: An Australian study, *Journal of Alternative and Complementary Medicine*, **12(7)**, 695–700.

Hamre, H., Becker-Witt, C., Glockmann, A., Ziegler, R., Willich, S., and Kiene, H. (2004). Anthroposophic therapies in chronic disease: The Anthroposophic Medicine Outcomes Study (AMOS), *European Journal of Medical Research*, **9(7)**, 351–360.

Herman, P., Sherman, K., Erro, J., Cherkin, D., Milliman, B., and Adams, L. (2006). A method for describing and evaluating naturopathic whole practice, *Alternative Therapies in Health and Medicine*, **12(4)**, 20–28.

Horrocks, S., Anderson, E., and Salisbury, C. (2002). Systematic review of whether nurse practitioners working in primary care can provide equivalent care to doctor, *British Medical Journal*, **324**, 819–823.

Hough, H., Dower, C., and O'Neil, E. (2001). *Profile of a Profession: Naturopathic Practice*, Center for the Health Professions, University of California, Berkeley.

Lin, V., Bensoussan, A., Myers, S., McCabe, P., Cohen, M., Hill, S., and Howse, G. (2005). *The Practice and Regulatory Requirements of Naturopathy and Western Herbal Medicine*, Department of Human Services, Melbourne.

Ma, J., Urizar, G.G., Alehegn, T., and Stafford, R. (2004). Diet and physical activity counseling during ambulatory care visits in the United States, *Preventive Medicine*, **39(4)**, 815–822.

Macinko, J., Starfield, B., and Shi, L. (2007). Quantifying the health benefits of primary care physician supply in the United States, *International Journal of Health Services*, **37(1)**, 111–126.

Nahin, R.L., Dahlhamer, J.M., Taylor, B., Barnes, P., Stussman, S., Simile, C., Blackman, M., Chesney, M., Jackson, M., Miller, H., and McFann, K. (2007). Health behaviors and risk factors in those who use complementary and alternative medicine, *BMC Public Health*, **7**, 217.

Naylor, M. and Kurtzman, E. (2010). The role of nurse practitioners in reinventing primary care, *Health Affairs*, **29(5)**, 893–899.

Nugent, R. (2008). Chronic diseases in developing countries: Health and economic burdens, *Annals of the New York Academy of Sciences*, **1136**, 70–79.

Parker, M., Wardle, J., Weir, M., and Stewart, C. (2011). Medical merchants: Conflict of interest, office product sales and notifiable conduct, *Medical Journal of Australia*, **194(1)**, 34–37.

Robert Graham Center. (2005). Osteopathic physicians and the family medicine workforce, *American Family Physician*, **72(4)**, 583.

Sarris, J. and Wardle, J. (eds.) (2010). *Clinical Naturopathy: An Evidence Based Guide to Practice*, Elsevier, Sydney.

Schneeweiss, R., Cherkin, D., Hart, L., Revicki, D., Wollstadt, L., Stephenson, M., Froom, J., Dunn, E., Tindall, H., and Rosenblatt, R. (1986). Diagnosis clusters adapted for ICD-9-CM and ICH-2, *Journal of Family Practice*, **22(1)**, 69–72.

Smith, C., Martin, K., Hotham, E., Semple, S., Bloustien, G., and Roa, D. (2005). Naturopaths practice behaviour: Provision and access to information on complementary and alternative medicines, *BMC Complementary and Alternative Medicine*, **5**, 15.

Stange, K. (2002). The paradox of the parts and the whole in understanding the and improving general practice, *International Journal of Quality in Health Care*, **14(4)**, 267–268.

Stange, K. (2009). The generalist approach, *Annals of Family Medicine*, **7(3)**, 198–203.

Stange, K. (2010). Power to advocate for health, *Annals of Family Medicine*, **8(2)**, 100–107.

Stange, K., Zyzanski, S., Jaén, C., Callahan, E., Kelly, R., Gillanders, W., Shank, J., Chao, J., Medalie, J., Miller, W., Crabtree, B., Flocke, S., Gilchrist, V., Langa D., and Goodwin, M. (1998). Illuminating the 'black box'. A description of 4,454 patient visits to 138 family physicians, *Journal of Family Practice*, **46(5)**, 377–389.

Starfield, B., Shi, L., and Macinko, J. (2005). Contribution of primary care to health systems and health, *Milbank Quarterly*, **83**, 457–502.

Steinsbekk, A., Rise, M., and Aickin, M. (2009). Cross-cultural comparison of visitors to CAM practitioners in the United States and Norway, *Journal of Alternative and Complementary Medicine*, **15(11)**, 1201–1207.

Tolhurst, H., Adams, J., and Stewart, S. (2006). An exploration of when urban background medical students become interested in rural practice, *International Journal of Remote and Rural Health,* **6(1)**, 452.

Tovey, P. and Adams, J. (2001). Primary care as intersecting social worlds, *Social Science and Medicine*, **52**, 695–706.

United States Department of Health and Human Services (2012). Loan repayment program for repayment of health professions educational loans; announcement type: Initial, *Federal Register*, **7(14)**, 3269–3272.

Verhoef, M., Boon, H., and Mutasingwa, D. (2006). The scope of naturopathic medicine in Canada: An emerging profession, *Social Science and Medicine*, **63(2)**, 409–417.

Victorian Parliament Joint Select Committee (1975). *Report from the Osteopathy, Chiropractic and Naturopathy Committee, together with appendices*, Government Printer, Melbourne.

Wardle, J., Adams, J., and Lui, C. (2010). A qualitative study of naturopathy in rural practice: A focus upon naturopaths' experiences and perceptions of rural patients and demands for their services, *BMC Health Services Research*, **10**, 185.

Wardle, J., Adams, J., Soares Magalhães, R., and Sibbritt, D. (2011). The distribution of complementary and alternative medicine (CAM) providers in rural New South Wales, Australia: A step towards explaining high CAM use in rural health? *Australian Journal of Rural Health*, **19(4)**, 197–204.

Wardle, J. and Oberg, E. (2011). The intersecting paradigms of naturopathic medicine and public health: Opportunities for naturopathic medicine, *Journal of Alternative and Complementary Medicine*, **17(11)**, 1079–1084.

Wardle, J., Steel, A., and Adams, J. (2012a). A review of tensions and risks in naturopathic education and training in Australia: A need for regulation, *Journal of Alternative and Complementary Medicine*, **18(40)**, 363–370.

Wardle, J., Lui, C., and Adams, J. (2012b). Complementary and alternative medicine in rural communities: Current research and future directions, *Journal of Rural Health*, **28(1)**, 101–112.

Wardle, J. and Adams, J. (2012). "The indirect risks of traditional, complementary and integrative medicine", in Adams, J., Andrews, G., Barnes, J., Magin, P., and Broom, A. (eds.), *Traditional, Complementary and Integrative Medicine: An International Reader*, Palgrave Macmillan, London, pp. 212–219.

Webb, E. (1977). *Report of the Committee of Inquiry into Chiropractic, Osteopathy, Homoeopathy and Naturopathy*, Australian Government Publishing Service, Canberra.

White House Commission on Complementary and Alternative Medicine Policy (2002). *United States of America White House Commission on Complementary and Alternative Medicine Policy Final Report*, Washington, DC.

Whorton, J. (2004). *Nature Cures: The History of Alternative Medicine in America*, Oxford University Press, New York.

Xue, C., Zhang, A., Lin, V., Da Costa, C., and Story, D. (2007). Complementary and alternative medicine use in Australia: A national population-based survey, *Journal of Alternative and Complementary Medicine*, **13(6)**, 643–650.

Zeff, J., Snider, P., and Myers, S. (2008). "A heirarchy of healing: The therapeutic order", in Pizzorno, J. and Murray, M. (eds.), *The Unifying Theory of Naturopathic Medicine. Textbook of Natural Medicine*, Elsevier, Philadelphia, pp. 27–40.

CHAPTER 5

Linking Complementary and Alternative Medicine, Traditional Medicine and Primary Health Care: The Role of Local Health Traditions in Promoting Health Security

Daniel Hollenberg and Maria Costanza Torri

5.1 Introduction

The field of complementary and alternative medicine (CAM) and integrative medicine (IM) can generally be considered as a global health phenomena (Hollenberg and Muzzin, 2010; Adams *et al.*, 2009; 2012). Within what can be termed "Western" or rich, industrialized health care systems, various CAM practices and systems have professionalized themselves alongside the medical profession, in a 150-year political tug of war characterized by the rise and relative fall of medical dominance and the legitimization of non-biomedical healing practices (Tovey *et al.*, 2004). CAM professions originated in both Europe (e.g., homeopathy) and North America (e.g., chiropractic and naturopathy) and also from traditional and indigenous health practices in non-Western countries (e.g., Chinese medicine). An inherent and often overlooked relationship was thus born between CAM in rich Western nations and traditional medicine (TM) — known to provide primary health care (PHC) to approximately 80% of citizens in poorer areas of the world — in non-Western countries. The rising popularity of CAM over the last 40 years can be paralleled by the development of TM policy in the World Health

93

Organization (WHO) within the same time frame (WHO, 2002; 2008). Moreover, in Western countries, IM reflects the combination of TM with conventional PHC campaigns in non-Western countries, a similarity that is often overlooked.

This chapter examines and critically reviews the widespread use of TM and its application to PHC in non-Western health care systems. Historically speaking, TM can be interpreted as the first or "original" form of CAM and PHC that has been practised for 5,000 years or more (Unschuld, 1998; 2009); drawing on a case study of "local health traditions" (LHT) in the form of home herbal gardens (HHG), this chapter offers a glimpse into the "real life" application of TM to address PHC concerns.

5.2 Overview of TM and PHC

It is important to clarify the differences between *traditional* medicine and *complementary/alternative* medicine. TM refers to long-standing indigenous systems of health care found mostly in developing countries and among the indigenous populations of industrialized countries. In these cultural settings individuals and the social collective are seen as more directly linked with nature and the environment on a day-to-day basis (than in non-indigenous cultures), knowledge is often passed down orally through generations and the focus is often upon restoring balance to body, mind and society (Bodeker, 2006). As Bodeker *et al.* further explain:

> In most developing countries, traditional health systems are grounded in long-standing cultural and spiritual values. Traditional health knowledge extends to an appreciation of both the material and non-material properties of plants, animals and minerals. Its classificatory systems range in scope from the cosmological to the particular, in addressing the physiological makeup of individuals and the specific categories of *material medica* (the materials used for therapeutic purposes) needed to enhance health and well-being. Mental, social, spiritual, physical and ecological factors are all taken into account (Bodeker *et al.*, 2007, p. 11).

Although clearly related, CAM refers to systems of health care distinct from biomedicine that are practised in rich, "developed" nations and may or may not include systems or parts of TM. For example, traditional Chinese medicine (TCM) is the TM system in China; however, TCM and/or acupuncture (a part of TCM) are viewed as a type of CAM when practised in North America, the United Kingdom, Israel and Europe (Janz and Adams, 2011). Although many definitions of TM and CAM continue to be offered and often coexist, a clear distinction can be made here with regard to their differences. Further, health care modalities such as chiropractic, massage therapy, naturopathy and homeopathy, while related to TM, are clearly CAM systems. The majority of the discussion that follows will largely focus on TM in a non-Western health care setting, as it is TM in particular that has been most overlooked in global health (Hollenberg *et al.*, 2012), mainly due to the observation that TM is not equitably included in international development initiatives (Pigg, 1995).

As Bodeker (2006) states, the use of TM can be thought of as responding to two fundamental questions: (i) how can countries address the health needs of their people without continuing to rely on expensive, imported medicines? and (ii) how can local, existing systems of health care be utilized to provide basic health services to rural and poor communities? A now often-cited statistic is that up to 80% of citizens in non-Western countries use some type of TM for direct PHC needs (although this figure would of course vary country by country) (Bodeker, 2006). For example, approximately 60% of individuals with HIV/AIDS in sub-Saharan Africa use TM (UNAIDS, 2000). The range of TM modalities includes herbal medicines (all forms), physical therapy and other body practices (e.g., massage and acupuncture), meditation, spiritual practices and strategies contributing to health promotion and prevention (e.g., women's health, birthing practices and midwifery). TM also has an extremely wide application, as demonstrated by the indigenous Aboriginal population of North America, who historically used over 500 medicinal plants to treat such illnesses as wounds, skin eruptions, stomach complaints, coughs/colds/fever, rheumatism/arthritis, freezing/frostbite, burns, cancer, blood poisoning, toothaches and others (Clark, 2004). Contemporary Aboriginal health care practices in North America continue to use surviving TM knowledge in the form of herbal and other medicinal practices.

Traditional medical knowledge, related practices and experiences are also partially defined by the social and cultural contexts in which they occur (Etkin and Elisabetsky, 2005; Godoy *et al.*, 2000). Traditional medical systems are embedded in local communities and vary from community to community according to structure and organization of the society. All cultures have shared ideas of what makes people sick, what cures them of these ailments and how they can maintain good health through time (Capuccio *et al.*, 2001). This cognitive development is part of the cultural heritage of each population, and from it empirical medical systems have been formed, based on the use of natural resources.

TM in particular has a long history in precolonial indigenous nations of treating a wide array of PHC concerns, extending from first-aid-type treatment for broken bones and burns to treatment for acute physical symptoms associated with infectious diseases such as diarrhoea (Bodeker and Burford, 2007). Much TM knowledge was lost through the direct actions of colonial powers that banned the use of TM in the nineteenth and twentieth centuries when Western medicine was professionalizing and expanding globally (e.g., Ayurvedic medicine was banned in nineteenth century India — see Banerji, 1981). Yet numerous TM traditions and a great deal of health knowledge have been re-established and are now essential aspects of health care systems in their countries of origin. For example, in countries such as China, India, Vietnam, Japan, Korea, Nepal, Thailand and various countries in Africa (e.g., Ghana), significant aspects of TM are directly integrated at the level of the national health care system (see WHO, 2002). As will be discussed below, TM has provided and continues to provide direct forms of PHC to global communities. By drawing on local resources, TM also provides important care to communities with low physician-to-population ratios and for those with poor access to Western biomedicine (Torri, 2011a, 2011b).

The efficacy of TM can be interpreted in a number of different ways, depending on theoretical orientation and interpretations of legitimate and "illegitimate" knowledge (Hollenberg and Muzzin, 2010; Adams, 2008). The marginalization of TM also happens in a number of simultaneously occurring ways. TM is overlooked for its potential impact on global health or recognized in only a limited fashion. When biomedical results analyzing TM are produced, results are often presented in such a way that limits the way a TM modality could be used for efficacy (Bodeker and Burford, 2007). In the section that follows, we focus on the last category of biomedical forms of TM evidence that have been underused in international health to date. Following Waldram (2000) and Pigg (1995), we agree that biomedical TM evidence represents only one type of "evidence" which has been marginalized in international health projects, in addition to other evidence types which include different kinds of healing (from physical to spiritual levels). We have chosen the most biomedically amenable forms of TM evidence to highlight how in those cases where TM is actually "proven", it remains largely ignored. As Waldram argues:

> It is essential that we comprehend the empirical nature of these medical systems and escape the lingering bonds of the antiquated view that traditional medicine can only be understood in terms of religion, superstition, and magic (Waldram, 2000, p. 610).

For the purposes of our discussion, the main strengths of TM that have been overlooked in the context of global health can be generally categorized into two main areas: (i) direct symptom management and reversal of acute diseases, and (ii) health promotion, management and prevention related to illness and disease and maintaining well-being. As noted, these two related strengths of TM can be viewed as an integral part of PHC in which TM is used to treat between 60% and 80% of the global burden of disease (Bodeker, 2006; Kaboru *et al.*, 2006).

5.3 TM and Primary Healthcare: A Case Study of Home Herbal Gardens (HHG)

Home herbal gardens (HHG) refer to one aspect of local health traditions employed in both urban, rural and usually non-Western communities where, worldwide, thousands of medicinal plants are grown for local use at the residential level (Torri and Hollenberg, 2011). The main types of health problems that can be addressed with HHG include cold, cough, fever, diarrhoea and dysentery, cuts, wounds, insect bites and women's reproductive health (e.g., dysmenorrhoea).

HHG are viewed as essential components of TM and PHC. For example, in parts of India, Hariramamurthi *et al.* (2007) report that a typical PHC centre servicing 30,000 local community citizens receives only

30,000 rupees per year, averaging only one rupee per year for each person who may attend the centre. In contrast to this paucity of biomedically based PHC, Hariramamurthi *et al.* note that:

> In India, Local Health Traditions (LHT) exist in rural communities. There are hundreds of millions of households and more than a million village healers who know about the use of ecosystem resources of plants, animals and minerals for human, veterinary and plant health. It has been documented that in India, 4,635 ethnic communities, including one million folk healers, use around 8,000 species of medicinal plants (Hariramamurthi *et al.*, 2007, p. 169).

Select HHG programmes have been initiated in various parts of India and now reach more than 6,000 villages and hamlets, with approximately 150,000 of these gardens in operation (Hariramamurthi *et al.*, 2007). Establishment of HHG programmes includes a participatory community and health care provider approach that invites community members and traditional and biomedical health providers (HPs) to pool their evaluative knowledge of effective medicinal plants in the community. Qualitative and quantitative evaluations have revealed that HHG are used largely by women, children and the elderly in extremely poor communities as effective responses to cough, cold and fever (Hariramamurthi *et al.*, 2007; Torri and Hollenberg, 2011). In addition to being effective, these gardens have also proven economical and accessible and, as such, contribute to poverty alleviation by reducing community health expenditures on foreign drugs and health care services (Torri and Laplante, 2009). As one example, it is evident that the cultivation of the raw herb *Artemesia annua* for malaria could easily be implemented through the HHG framework; to date, this TCM herb is known globally to be the most effective treatment for malaria over and above its synthetic drug equivalent, artemisinin (Bodeker and Burford, 2007).

The concept of HHG was first formulated in Bangalore and Tamil Nadu, South India, through the Foundation for the Revitalization of Local Health Traditions (FRLHT), a non-profit non-governmental organization (NGO) founded in 1993 (in the Southern Indian state of Karnataka). The FRLHT was established in the early 1990s to revitalize Indian local health

traditions through a range of field activities, research and extension programmes focused on conserving TM in various rural communities of
South India. As Torri and Laplante (2009) have noted, the FRLHT has
extensively documented TM in relation to medicinal plants, and further,
the enhancement of local capacity building through workshops and
courses targeted to rural communities in South India. Very few NGOs are
currently engaged in the protection of TM knowledge for promoting and
enhancing PHC (Torri and Laplante, 2009). The three main goals of the
FRLHT are: (i) conservation of natural resources used by TM systems, (ii)
demonstration of the contemporary relevance of the theory and practice
linked to TM and (iii) revitalization of the social processes (institutional,
rural and commercial) to ensure transmission of traditional knowledge.

As Torri and Laplante (2009) note, the extensive use of HHG as a form
of TM can be specifically conceptualized as engaging the important concept of "ethnomedicine capacity" — a combination of interactions between
scientific members and researchers of the FRLHT, and specific community
members and folk healers from the various community outreach programmes that the FRLHT facilitates. Ethnomedicine capacity also involves
the combination of research and action, and consists of the documentation
and conservation of medicinal plants, the dissemination of knowledge and
the increase of awareness among villagers and community members regarding the use of TM practices. The FRLHT has extensively focused on participatory research with local South Indian communities in order to identify
specific medicinal plants traditionally used by community members.

In the first year of FRLHT's activities, the foundation documented
extensive information related to health practices, remedies and local species of medicinal plants used to treat a variety of health conditions.
According to a nomenclature database developed by the FRLHT, there are
approximately 50,000 local names relating to roughly 4,800 medicinal
plants used in the context of TM. Within the HHG context, the FRLHT
further documented the knowledge of approximately 200 TM practitioners, of which 31 were traditional birth attendants (TBAs). In total, approximately 578 medicinal formulas have been recorded. The Foundation also
documented that HHG, as an aspect of TM, are primarily related to the oral
transmission of a traditional "folk" healing system practised by specific
village physicians (also called folk healers) within the tribal communities

of South India. These specific folk systems were related to, but also distinctly different from, the more formal systems of TM in India, such as Ayurveda, Sidha and Unani TM systems. In contrast to folk systems related to HHG, the more formal TM Indian systems listed above are based on organized, codified and synthesized medical wisdom with strong theoretical and conceptual foundations as well as philosophical explanations (Torri and Laplante, 2009).

In addition to the health and medicinal aspects of specific TM plants, information was also collected on the socio-economic and ethnocultural aspects that are inherently connected with the practice of HHG. For example, approximately 600 women in 400 households from 60 villages were interviewed to record specific household remedies associated with medicinal plants, alongside the documentation of more than 700 specific healing practices. Furthermore, the FRLHT documented specific pharmacological standards for 61 plants with the help of local folk healers. The Foundation has also been involved in the documentation and standardization of plant extracts in conjunction with folk healers using conventional techniques and models.

In conjunction with local communities, the FRLHT has further developed the Community Health Traditions Register (CHTR), specifically created for the protection of community intellectual property rights. Participatory workshops have been offered to various interested communities, where community members work to identify and document the main medicinal plants, the economic significance for ecological history as well as information related to indigenous and local community lands and territories. The inspiration for the CHTR arose partially from a desire to protect community intellectual property rights and also from a community desire to renew and develop resource management strategies led by local villagers. As part of protecting intellectual property rights, the FRLHT specializes in developing needs-based training courses and educational events as a way of supporting the process of preserving and revitalizing what can be termed "Indian medical heritage."

In the context of protecting and revitalizing Indian medical heritage, a conservation park of medicinal plants was developed in the Nadurai district on a specific campus named Sevayoor (Torri and Laplante, 2009). The overarching goal of the conservation park is to further educate villagers and to increase their knowledge of medicinal plants and traditional health practices. The park consists of an ethnomedicine forest spanning 33 acres and boasting a collection of more than 500 plant species. The park could be perceived, from a Western health systems perspective, as one of the most unique and original aspects of the HHG concept. The park operates as an open space where local villagers, other communities and students can interact and participate with all aspects of medicinal plants specifically grown in the South Indian geographical zone. Sevayoor also houses a medicinal plant dispensary as well as a medicinal preparation unit under the supervision of several traditional folk healers living and/or residing on campus. Further, two specific village organizations manage the medicinal plant dispensary and also prepare medicines for the community and surrounding area.

As noted above, various research studies have been conducted via the FRLHT on different aspects related to HHG. One specific study was conducted in conjunction with several local village organizations in order to analyze changes in community health, food regime and routine, and the ability to manage medicinal needs in the context of evaluating community participation. This specific study showed that in poor households, health expenses were high and rural women had very little access to resources such that their own health was a last priority within the household. In response to these findings, a community-based enterprise was created to promote and maintain sustainable cultivation and utilization of medicinal plants, and to educate community members on the importance of using TM-based plants for their basic PHC needs. The training programmes that resulted from the community enterprise further helped women to recognize and value local knowledge in the form of medicinal plants. What is fascinating is that the community enterprise now provides livelihood opportunities to over 1,200 families who are mostly landless labourers in over 160 village organizations, and 400 families of small- and medium-sized property farmers. This has directly enhanced the health of the participating communities (Torri, 2011a, 2011b). This community-based enterprise active in the herbal sector is not only limited to the sale of phytomedicines, however. Following the training that villagers have received, women are able to play the role of consultant for basic health needs *vis-à-vis* other women in the community.

As Torri (2010) has documented, community-based enterprises associ-ated with TM in South India have been successful in producing an enhanced social status for participating women. Although not directly related to PHC, the involvement of women in TM-based enterprises has contributed to an increase in women's access to power and resources at both community and household levels. The empowerment of communities and women in particular, is nevertheless an important aspect of PHC as empowerment leads to increased social status, which in turn has a direct correlation with increased health status. Mr Hariramamurthi, one of the key programme officers at the FRLHT, argues that Indian folk traditions are ethnic-community and ecosystem-specific (personal communication, 2010). Mr Hariramamurthi clarifies that biodiversity and cultural diversity are inherently connected and "go hand in hand"; he argues that local health traditions and biodiversity of medicinal plants are very critical for the health security of the rural and urban populations who are not covered by conventional government, private or non-government health care sec-tors. He also clarifies that local health traditions, distinct and different from formal codified health care systems in India, are practised at the household level to address basic PHC needs, including the use of diverse food recipes, seasonal regimens, customs and rituals (personal communi-cation, 2010). The "folk stream" aspect of local health traditions is part of the larger cultural routine including lifestyle, diet and health practices essential for literally thousands of local South Indian communities. It is Mr Hariramamurthi's hope that all HHG programmes will be integrated through PHC centres in South India.

5.4 Discussion

A significant observation that should be noted when discussing TM is that although widely used by millions of citizens globally, its use is not reflected or incorporated into the majority of government-funded interna-tional health campaigns initiated by Western or "rich" nations (Bodeker and Burford, 2007). This ongoing conservative biomedical policy can be traced to an exclusive reliance on biomedically-centred evidence models and, further, rests upon an epistemological bias against indigenous knowl-edge that has its origins in colonial thinking (Harding, 1998). Following the detailed work of anti/post-colonial scholars such as Harding (1998) and Shiva (1993, 1997), we consider the colonial view of TM as the major diagnostic problem leading to the current concept of TM in international/ global health programmes. As such anti/postcolonial scholars often note that valuable and legitimate ideas that originate in Southern countries often do not receive the attention they deserve in the global debate and are viewed with little confidence. Yet Southern ideas consistently retain the capacity to rebuild local patterns of development (Jentsch and Pilley, 2003).

Since 1978, TM has been recognized by the WHO as important for advances in global health and recent TM policy documents (e.g., WHO 2002; 2008) emphasize the role of TM in health care systems. At the same time, the main prevention approach advocated for major global diseases is increased access to biomedical forms of drug-based treatment, such as antiretroviral (ARV) drugs, not TM (Bodeker *et al.*, 2007). Critically informed anthropologists consistently question why the evidence and/or science of TM (such as HHG) is not included in international development policy and projects. As Pigg states:

> Often it is simply assumed, without seeking evidence, that only the medical solutions offered by development save lives, when, in fact, it remains a matter for research and debate just how "efficacy" is to be evaluated and what sorts of medical techniques and therapeutic systems, in precisely what kinds of social contexts, alleviate bodily suffering "best" (Pigg, 1995, p. 49).

As Kaboru *et al.* (2008) further comment, what remains to be resolved is how this consistent biomedical orientation to large-scale international health projects will operate in various non-Western countries, where biomedical health care is financially out of reach to many and where staff are in short supply, overwhelmed or simply non-existent. Physician-to-population ratios in many areas of the world are sometimes as low as one physician for every 100,000 citizens (Bodeker, 2006). As Pigg comments:

> Mainstream development programmes that work with indigenous knowledge ... manage the circulation of discourses in ways that ensure that development knowledge seems to count everywhere, while indigenous knowledge counts in only limited and carefully controlled ways (Pigg, 1995, p. 49).

In certain areas of health care policy (e.g., Homsy *et al.*, 2004; WHO, 1990; UNAIDS, 2000) TM is viewed as a targeted resource discussed as part of scaling up efforts to control disease such as HIV/AIDS and malaria. The main approach, continuing to reflect a biomedical bias toward TM, is to retrain traditional HPs to deliver biomedical PHC skills and services, such as public health education and counselling, and condom distribution in the case of HIV infections (see King, 1999; Peltzer *et al.*, 2006; UNAIDS, 2000). Although biomedical training for traditional HPs remains important, in the minority are new approaches that focus on biomedical HPs and traditional HPs learning together and from each other (see Kaboru *et al.*, 2006), and working together for the general health of their shared populations.

Even with focused efforts toward a more balanced approach to the professional interface between biomedical and traditional HPs, negative biomedical attitudes toward TM continue to surface among biomedical HPs, even in China, where TCM is protected by government policy and is a big part of shared tradition (Hollenberg and Muzzin, 2010). The anthropological debate on TM criticizes policies of integration between TM and biomedicine (Helman, 2007). Rance Lee (1982), recognizing the unequal relationship that generally characterizes the coexistence of various therapeutic traditions in a society, has studied therapeutic pluralism in terms of the domination of one medical tradition over another, what he calls *hierarchical pluralism.*

An optimistic argument has been proposed by some to suggest that the ongoing criticism by biomedical HPs working with traditional HPs reflects a critical awareness process full of conflict and tension, which it is hoped could adapt biomedical HPs to become reflective and capable of questioning their own assumptions and, also, become more open to new perspectives (Kaboru *et al.*, 2008, p. 121). In the profession's literature, biomedical HPs are naïvely portrayed as reacting from their perspective of strong professional values that are simply resistant to new perspectives (Hall, 2005), yet a more critical theoretical perspective suggests that the majority of biomedical HPs have absorbed an ingrained bias against non-reductionist knowledge (Harding, 1998).

This chapter argues that, historically and currently, the role of TM has consistently been overlooked and/or neglected in global health initiatives, despite the above-stated strengths that include direct treatment of infectious diseases and health promotion/disease prevention strategies. Arguably, the major reason for this lack of inclusion can be directly linked to an epistemological bias within biomedicine and Western science that ignores and/or devalues the worth of indigenous knowledge even when presenting evidence-based information. The devaluation of indigenous health knowledge has created a "conceptual gap", leaving the potential use of TM in global international health endeavours largely unaddressed. In this dualistic vision, health typologies are described primarily as Western or non-Western forms of knowledge, defined only in relation to the West. Such reductionism seeks to contain diverse genres of TM or non-Western knowledge in one undifferentiated category. As a consequence, aspects of typology, instrumental action, experimentation, logical thinking, individualism and causality are assumed to only occur in Western science (Greenhalgh and Wessely, 2004; Hernández, 2003; Kaptchuk and Eisenberg, 2001; Harding, 1998).

Although WHO documents have possibly expanded the awareness of TM in the international health community, the response to TM that can be viewed in the international biomedical health literature continues to reflect a reductionist biomedical bias (Hollenberg and Muzzin, 2010; Harding, 1998). Moreover, it is fair to say that the majority of policy issues involving TM as endorsed by the WHO have yet to be widely implemented by international health projects "on the ground", also a likely symptom of the continued biomedical bias against TM. This lack of engagement can be repeatedly observed even with the renewed emphasis on TM by new leaders in the WHO; while stating that "traditional medicine can also help prevent so-called modern lifestyle diseases such as diabetes, heart disease and mental disorders", WHO leaders insist that "many traditional medicines have an inadequate evidence base when measured by these [biomedical] standards" (Schearf, 2008). Health researchers around the world who are working directly with TM in HIV/AIDS patient populations, for example, are frustrated with this contradictory agenda (see Kaboru *et al.*, 2006).

It should be noted that attempts to measure efficacy of TM using Randomized Controlled Trials (RCT) and other forms of scientific assessment, which are highly ranked in the hierarchy of evidence, are philosophically and theoretically problematic (Adams, 2002; Adams *et al.*, 2005; Borgerson, 2005; Barry, 2005; Villanueva-Russell, 2004; Goldenberg, 2006). Philosophically, the reductionist characteristic of positivist epistemology, that underpins biomedicine's view of efficacy and focuses on the removal of symptoms and diseases, is too narrow to evaluate TM, which deals not only with disease but also with holistically affective, social and spiritual well-being. Although new reductionist designs are attempted, theoretical differences in knowledge about human anatomy and physiology, disease etiology, classification and diagnosis between biomedicine and other medical systems entail different sets of definitions and measurements of effectiveness as well as criteria for evaluating success. For instance, many studies have observed a distinction between epistemologies that underpin biomedicine and Asian medical systems. Unschuld (1987) insists that epistemological differences between Indian (South Asian) and Western medicine actually lie in the differences in attitudes toward truth, or what he calls "patterned knowledge between Indian knowledge and Western mono-paradigmatic science".

Within the pervasive conservative biomedical tradition that has invaded international health policymaking, TM is viewed colonially as a resource only to be cautiously explored for its potential benefit to increase the effectiveness of biomedical PHC techniques. From the biomedical perspective, the inherent challenge of TM is how to use a valuable resource while attempting to tame or restrict its "wild", uncontrollable qualities (such as perceived side effects and the misguidance of patients to ineffective treatments). Biomedical critics of TM are quick to query if TM can treat infectious diseases like malaria and HIV/AIDS, why has there not been an eradication of these diseases worldwide? The main response to this critique is that while TM is certainly not a cure-all for infectious disease and while drugs are certainly important, TM *can* have efficacy in locally embedded contexts (Bodeker and Burford, 2007). At the same time, however, the widespread therapeutic effect of local knowledge has been marginalized through colonization, with the overall consequence that TM is undervalued in biomedical and international health communities (Harding, 1998). The extensive network of HHG documented in this chapter is a case-in-point, as this overlooked local PHC model clearly provides care to millions of citizens but has yet to be acknowledged by the WHO.

The inherent biomedical bias against TM has additional consequences that directly affect relationships between patients, TM and biomedical HPs. Just as with CAM in more industrialized nations, patients using TM are hesitant to disclose their use of TM when consulting a biomedical HP, such as in more formal PHC clinics. Historically, relations between biomedical and traditional HPs have been strained, with little communication and cross-referral, similar to tensions between biomedical HPs and CAM providers. There also exist significant clinical consequences of poor communication between TM and biomedical HPs, most notably potential adverse events between modalities and lack of recognition of efficacy and contextual practice of TM.

5.5 Conclusion

Although an attempt to reposition TM as an essential health resource in international health faces many challenges, it is useful to consider a different approach that might be taken in the future. We propose that, at the outset, TM must be considered as legitimate and coherent systems of locally embedded healing knowledge with relevance to the local communities in which it is used. Although this stance does not preclude its wider application to global populations (e.g., the use of the TCM herb *Artemesia* for malaria), TM can be most effectively used at the community level in which it originated and is practised. While TM is certainly not a panacea, substantial areas of health and wellness can be maintained with its use, as noted above. TM also has the inherent strength of being able to work with, or alongside, other health measures, and does not need to be altered by a biomedical agenda. For example, modified and culturally sensitive public health measures such as clean water, effective housing, shelter and access to viable food sources all contribute to an ecological system that promotes the efficacy of TM and the health of communities in which it is practised. Evidence already exists demonstrating that when TM is altered and/or synthesized for its component parts, not only does it become less effective, it also contradicts the bioethical tenet of non-maleficence by causing increased harm in patient populations (that is, increased side effects and/or pathogen resistance, such as within the synthetic drug *artemisinin* for malaria) (Bodeker and Burford, 2007). Viewing TM as both legitimate and clinically effective health knowledge repositions TM in ways in which it has not previously been widely viewed. This perspective moves past the purely ethnographic viewpoint which classifies TM as a cultural practice without clinical benefit and re-conceptualizes TM as having a healing benefit, and not only as a vehicle for biomedical retraining.

The most effective approach for an equitable view of TM could be to forge partnerships between traditional HPs who practise TM and biomedical HPs associated with international PHC projects. Policymakers such as Kaboru *et al.* (2006) have already imagined how partnerships could operate, despite these professional patterns of interaction having yet to be implemented in many areas of the world. For example, Kaboru *et al.* argue for the clinical education of *both* traditional and biomedical HPs in each other's basic knowledge and/or respective paradigms in a manner that does not detract or demote the knowledge of traditional HPs, nor provide biomedical HPs a monopoly over patient care. Modified degrees of international policy intervention could also be implemented to recognize when an operational TM system requires little or no assistance from biomedical PHC and when biomedical HPs could be useful, based on community input. Many of these challenges and scenarios mirror developments in IM in Western societies where biomedical and CAM practitioners are working together in the same clinic (see Hollenberg, 2006; 2007). Although far from resolving the above challenges, IM in more industrialized health care settings and countries has identified ideals, although perhaps utopian, including trust, respect and establishing a seamless continuum of care. Thus, a theory exists for integration between divergent modalities that could be applied to the interaction between TM and PHC campaigns (Hollenberg and Bourgeault, 2011).

It should also be re-emphasized that a handful of countries, as pointed out by the WHO, have longstanding systems of TM and biomedicine that already work alongside each other and are at times approaching patterns of integration. For example, China has fully functional TCM-Western IM hospitals. Though there are advances here, even China has not escaped the effect of biomedical marginalization of TCM (see Unschuld, 1998; Scheid, 2002), pointing to the need to reposition TM as essential knowledge. In China, TCM knowledge is becoming viewed as inferior to Western science and technology and TCM researchers are being encouraged to modify their research designs so that their research may be published in Western scientific journals (D. Cai, personal communication, 2007).

In summary, future TM policy should take into account the following: (i) TM must be evaluated using its own internally coherent systems of healing knowledge, in the context of community-level interventions, without being altered by biomedical techniques or theory that would make the TM system unrecognizable by the respective TM practitioner, (ii) TM must be recognized as clinically effective and providing pragmatic health benefits, in addition to its important symbolic and cultural meaning, all of which are linked and, at times, inseparable, (iii) traditional and biomedical HPs need to work together in a way that does not devalue and/or alter the inherent worth and clinical benefit of TM knowledge and does not give biomedical HPs a monopoly over patients when PHC campaigns are implemented and (iv) wide-scale TM policy initiatives at institutional and governmental levels need to recognize the above, and the ongoing deleterious effect of Western science on indigenous and/or traditional healing knowledge.

References

Adams, J. (2008). *Researching Complementary and Alternative Medicine*, Routledge, London.

Adams, J., Hollenberg, D., Broom, A., and Lui, C. (2009). Contextualising integration: A critical social science approach to integrative healthcare, *Journal of Manipulative and Physiological Therapeutics*, **32(9)**, 792–798.

Adams, J., Andrews, G., Barnes, J., Broom, A., and Magin, P. (eds.) (2012). *Traditional, Complementary and Integrative Medicine: An International Reader*, Palgrave, London.

Adams, V. (2002). Randomized controlled crime: Postcolonial sciences in alternative medicine research, *Social Studies of Science*, **32(5/6)**, 659–690.

Adams, V., Miller, S., Craig, S., Nyima, S., Droyoung, L., and Varner, M. (2005). The challenge of cross-cultural clinical trials research: Case report from the Tibetan autonomous region, People's Republic of China, *Medical Anthropology Quarterly*, **19(3)**, 267–289.

Banerji, D. (1981). The place of indigenous and Western systems of medicine in the health services of India, *Social Science and Medicine*, **15(A)**, 109–114.

Barry, C. A. (2006). The role of evidence in alternative medicine: Contrasting biomedical and anthropological approaches, *Social Science and Medicine*, **62(11)**, 2646–2657.

Bodeker, G. (2006). "Global dimensions", in Micozzi, S. (ed.), *Fundamentals of Complementary and Integrative Medicine*, Elsevier, St. Louis, pp. 82–92.

Bodeker, G. and Burford, G. (eds.) (2007). *Traditional, Complementary and Alternative Medicine: Policy and Public Health Perspectives*, Imperial College Press, London.

Bodeker, G., Kronenberg, F., and Burford, G. (2007). "Policy and public health perspectives on traditional, complementary and alternative medicine: An overview", in Bodeker, G. and Burford, G. (eds.), *Traditional, Complementary and Alternative Medicine: Policy and Public Health Perspectives*, Imperial College Press, London, pp. 9–40.

Borgerson, K. (2005). Evidence-based alternative medicine? *Perspectives in Biology and Medicine*, **48(4)**, 502–515.

Clark, J. (2004). *Health, Illness, and Medicine in Canada*, Oxford University Press, New York.

Capuccio, F. P., Duneclift, S. M., Atkinson, R. W., and Cook, D. G. (2001). Alternative medicines in a multi-ethnic population, *Ethnicity and Disease*, **1(1)**, 11–18.

Etkin, N. L. and Elisabetsky, E. (2005). Seeking a transdisciplinary and culturally germane science: The future of ethnopharmacology, *Journal of Ethnopharmacology*, **1(2)**, 23–26.

Godoy, R., Wilkie, D., Overman, H., Cubas, A., Cubas G., Demmer J., and Brokaw, N. (2000). Valuation of consumption and sale of forest goods from a Central American rain forest, *Nature*, **40(6)**, 62–63.

Goldenberg, M. J. (2006). On evidence and evidence-based medicine: Lessons from the philosophy of science, *Social Science and Medicine*, **62(11)**, 2621–2632.

Greenhalgh, T. and Wessely, S. (2004). "Health for me": A socio-cultural analysis of healthism in the middle classes, *British Medical Bulletin*, **6(9)**, 197–213.

Hall, P. (2005). Interprofessional teamwork: Professional cultures as barriers, *Journal of Interprofessional Care*, **19(1)**, 188–196.

Han, G. (2000). Traditional herbal medicine in the Korean community in Australia: A strategy to cope with health demands of migrant life, *Health*, **4(2)**, 426–454.

Harding, S. (1998). *Is Science Multicultural? Postcolonialisms, Feminisms, and Epistemologies*, Indiana University Press, Bloomington.

Hariramamurthi, G., Venkatasubramian, P., Unnikrishnan, P. M., and Shankar, D. (2007). "Home herbal gardens: A novel health security strategy based on local knowledge and resources", in Bodeker, G. and Burford, G. (eds.), *Traditional Complementary and Alternative medicine: Policy and Public Health Perspectives*, Imperial College Press, London, pp. 167–184.

Helman, C. G. (2007). *Culture, Health and Illness*, Hodder Arnold, London.

Hernández, I. (2003). *Autonomía o ciudadanía incompleta. El pueblo mapuche en Chile y Argentina*, CEPAL — Pehuén Eds, Santiago.

Hobson, H. L. (2006). Sexual magic and money: Miskitu women's strategies in Northern Honduras, *Ethnology*, **45(2)**, 143–159.

Hollenberg, D. (2006). Uncharted ground: Patterns of professional interaction among complementary/alternative and biomedical practitioners in integrative healthcare settings, *Social Science and Medicine*, **62**, 731–744.

Hollenberg, D. (2007). How do private CAM therapies affect integrative health-care settings in a publicly funded healthcare system? *Journal of Complementary and Integrative Medicine*, **4(1)**.

Hollenberg, D. and Muzzin, L. (2010). Epistemological challenges to integrative medicine: An anti-colonial perspective on the combination of complementary/alternative medicine with biomedicine, *Health Sociology Review*, **19(1)**, 34–56.

Hollenberg, D. and Bourgeault, I. (2011). Linking integrative medicine with interprofessional education and care initiatives: Challenges and opportunities for interprofessional collaboration, *Journal of Interprofessional Care*, **25**, 182–188.

Hollenberg, D., Zakus, D., Cook, T., and Xu X. W. (2012). "Repositioning the role of traditional medicine as essential health knowledge in global health: Do they still have a role to play?", in Adams, J., Andrews, G., Barnes, J., Broom, A., and Magin, P. (eds.), *Traditional, Complementary and Integrative Medicine: An International Reader*, Palgrave, London, pp. 237–244.

Homsy, J., King, R., Balaba, D., and Kabatesi, D. (2004). Traditional health practitioners are key to scaling up comprehensive care for HIV/AIDS in sub-Saharan Africa, *AIDS*, **18**, 1723–1725.

Janz, S. and Adams, J. (2011). Acupuncture education standards in Australia: A critical review, *Australian Journal of Acupuncture and Chinese Medicine*, **6(1)**, 3–15.

Jentsch, B. and Pilley, C. (2003). Research relationships between the south and the north: Cinderella and the ugly sisters? *Social Science and Medicine*, **57**, 1957–1967.

Kaboru, B.B., Falkenberg, T., Ndubani, P., Höjer, B., Vongo, R., Brugha, R., and Faxelid, E. (2006). Can biomedical and traditional healthcare providers work together? Zambian practitioners' experiences and attitudes towards collaboration in relation to STIs and HIV/AIDS care: A cross-sectional study, *Human Resources for Health*, **4(16)**, 1–8.

Kaboru, B.B., Ndubani, P., Falkenberg, T., Pharris, A., Muchimba, M., Solo, K., and Höjer, B. (2008). A dialogue-building pilot intervention involving traditional and biomedical health providers focusing on STIs and HIV/AIDS care in Zambia, *Complementary Health Practice Review*, **13(2)**, 110–126.

Kaptchuk, T. and Eisenberg, D. (2001). Varieties of healing: Medical pluralism in the United States, *Annals of Internal Medicine*, **5(3)**, 189–195.

King, R. (1999). *Collaboration with traditional healers in AIDS prevention and care in sub-Saharan Africa: A comparative case study using UNAIDS best practice criteria*, UNAIDS, Geneva.

Lee, R.P. (1982). Comparative studies of health care systems, *Social Science and Medicine*, **16(6)**, 629–642.

Peltzer, K., Mngqundaniso, N., and Petros, G. (2006). A controlled study of a HIV/AIDS/STI/TB intervention with traditional healers in KwaZulu-Natal, South Africa, *AIDS Behaviour*, **10**, 683–690.

Pigg, S.L. (1995). Acronyms and effacement: Traditional medical practitioners (TMP) in international health development, *Social Science and Medicine*, **41(1)**, 47–68.

Schearf, D. (2008). WHO promotes Chinese model for integrated traditional medicine, *WHO Chinese Medicine Report*.

Scheid, V. (2002). *Chinese Medicine in Contemporary China: Plurality and Synthesis*, Duke University Press, Durham.

Shiva, V. (1993). *Monocultures of the Mind*, Zed Books, London.

Shiva, V. (1997). *Biopiracy: The Plunder of Nature and Knowledge*, South End Press, Boston.

Torri, M.C. (2010). Increasing knowledge and traditional use of medicinal plants by local communities in Tamil Nadu: Promoting self-reliance at the grass-roots level through a community-based entrepreneurship initiative, *Journal of Evidence-Based Complementary and Alternative Medicine*, **15(1)**, 40–51.

Torri, M.C. (2011a). Multicultural social policy and community participation in health: New opportunities and challenges for indigenous people, *International Journal of Health Planning and Management*, **26(3)**, 1–23.

Torri, M.C. (2011b). The importance of social capital in the promotion of community development and the enhancement of local health systems, *Journal of Health Management*, **13(1)**, 15–38.

Torri, M.C. and Laplante, J. (2009). Enhancing innovation between scientific and indigenous knowledge: Pioneer NGOs in India, *Journal of Ethnobiology and Ethnomedicine*, **5**, 29.

Torri, M.C. and Hollenberg, D. (2011). Therapeutic uses of edible plants in Bangalore city, India: Combining health with cooking practices through home herbal gardens, *Environment, Development and Sustainability*, **14(3)**, 303–319.

Tovey, P., Easthope, G., and Adams, J. (eds.) (2004). *The Mainstreaming of Complementary and Alternative Medicine: Studies in Social Context*, Routledge, London.

UNAIDS (2000). Collaboration with traditional healers in HIV/AIDS prevention and care in Sub-Saharan Africa: A literature review, *UNAIDS Best Practice Collection, Joint United Nations Programme on AIDS*, UNAIDS, Geneva.

Unschuld, P. U. (1987). Traditional Chinese medicine: Some historical and epistemological reflections, *Social Science and Medicine*, **24(12)**, 1023–1029.

Unschuld, P. (1998). *Chinese Medicine*, Paradigm Publications, Brookline.

Unschuld, P. (2009). *What is medicine? Western and Eastern Approaches to Healing*, University of California Press, Berkeley.

Villanueva-Russell, Y. (2005). Evidence-based medicine and its implications for the profession of chiropractic, *Social Science and Medicine*, **60**, 545–561.

Waldram, J.B. (2000). The efficacy of traditional medicine: Current theoretical and methodological issues, *Medical Anthropology Quarterly*, **14(4)**, 609–625.

WHO (1990). *Global Programme on AIDS and Traditional Medicine. Report of a WHO Consultation on Traditional Medicine and AIDS: Clinical Evaluation of Traditional Medicines and Natural Product*, WHO, Geneva.

WHO (2002). *Traditional medicine strategy 2002–2005*, WHO, Geneva.

WHO (2008). *Beijing Declaration*, WHO, Geneva.

CHAPTER 6

Examining the Relationship between Complementary and Integrative Medicine and Rural General Practice: A Focus upon Health Services Research

Jon Wardle, Jon Adams, Alex Broom, and David Sibbritt

6.1 Introduction

Recent research has revealed that complementary and integrative medicine (CIM) is particularly popular amongst rural populations, with a growing body of literature supporting this interpretation (Wardle *et al.*, 2012). Nevertheless, despite long-standing calls for further research in this area (Adams, 2004) very little is known about how, when and why primary health care (PHC) patients utilise CIM and even less is known about the grass-roots interface between CIM and conventional PHC in the context of rural health care.

This chapter draws upon existing literature and an emerging programme of research to examine and understand these features of rural health care delivery and consumption. The chapter also explores a number of issues of concern to rural general practitioners (GPs) on this topic and identifies the major research gaps in this area, as well as introducing some of the possible future work that may help to address such gaps.

6.1.1 *Complementary and integrative medicine in rural areas*

Recent international studies have highlighted different patterns of CIM utilisation across the rural–urban divide (Wardle *et al.*, 2012). In many cases, CIM use is higher in certain rural areas as compared with urban areas, with several factors underlying these different patterns of use. Such high use may be related to differential access to biomedical care and related health services, cultural norms and traditions of trust in complementary and alternative medicine (CAM) approaches to health care, lower income and health insurance in remote regions, and simply the high availability of CAM practitioners/practices in rural areas (Leipert and Reutter, 2005; McColl, 2007; Lind *et al.*, 2009; Wardle *et al.*, 2011; Zhang *et al.*, 2008; van der Weg and Streuli, 2003; Featherstone *et al.*, 2003; Barish and Snyder, 2008).

Additionally, specific cultural traits have been identified as driving CIM use amongst rural populations, including enhanced social capital, increased levels of spirituality, an affinity with holistic interpretations of health and attention to nutrition (Wardle *et al.*, 2010; Robinson and Chesters, 2008). This cultural connection may have even deeper roots — a qualitative exploration of Australian naturopaths' perceptions of high rural demand for their services suggested rural areas (and thereby rural populations) may hold a historical affinity for these therapies, as Australian naturopathy had been perceived to develop in rural parts of the country (Wardle *et al.*, 2010). This would also appear to mirror the rural roots of other CIM therapies such as chiropractic and osteopathy (Whorton, 2004).

The consumption of CIM in rural areas is a significant contemporary health care issue (Adams *et al.*, 2003). It has been widely reported that conventional health services are stretched in rural areas (Wilkinson *et al.*, 2004; Bradshaw *et al.*, 2006) and CIM may be able to provide, and in some cases is certainly already providing, a resource or network of care and provision for rural patients (Wardle *et al.*, 2012). There is also evidence that high-risk groups living in rural areas, such as older people and ethnic minorities, are frequent CIM users (Cuellar *et al.*, 2003; Arcury *et al.*, 2006; Ng *et al.*, 2006; Shreffler-Grant *et al.*, 2007). As such, an understanding of CIM use in rural health can provide a new perspective on health beliefs and practices as well as some of the core service delivery issues facing rural health care more generally.

There has been an emergence of a geographical perspective with regard to researching CIM, advancing a broad focus on the dynamics of well-being, health practices and spatial locations with regard to these medicines (Andrews, 2003; Andrews *et al.*, 2004; 2010; 2012; Gesler and Kearns, 2002; Hoyez, 2007). While such work has been of significance, especially with regard to theorising and conceptualising the role of CIM use and practice, it has not subjected the topic of CAM in rural health to in-depth or systematic investigation.

6.1.2 *CIM and rural general practice*

General practice is one branch of medicine where CIM has made its presence felt (Adams 2004b; Phelps and Hassed, 2011). General practitioners (GPs) and family practitioners or family physicians are regional terms for the same profession or specialisation of medicine. GPs will be used to refer to both family physicians/practitioners and general practitioners throughout this chapter for reasons of consistency. Rural GPs' perspectives and practices regarding CIM are particularly significant and influential for current rural health services and use (whether conventional or complementary in form) as well as the future exposure and location of CIM practice alongside rural conventional health care and the possible future role(s) of CIM practitioners in delivering health care to rural communities. These issues are made ever more pertinent by research that suggests high use of CIM by rural populations (Adams *et al.*, 2003; 2011; del Mundo *et al.*, 2002; Sherwood, 2000; Nunes and Sena Esteves, 2006; Wilkinson and Simpson, 2001).

GPs in rural communities often act as the primary or sole interface between medical and other health services and patients (Glasgow *et al.*, 2004). To some extent, this role may also be present in patient's interface between CIM and conventional medical practice, with research suggesting that conventional medical doctors are a preferred source of CIM information for a significant number of rural CIM users (Robinson, 2007).

However, to date few studies have focused on CIM as it relates to and interfaces with the conventional PHC workforce (such as GPs), with even fewer studies on PHC providers in rural areas. Those studies that have looked at PHC providers have focused on practitioner use or attitudes towards the personal use of CIM in their patient base rather than exploring the associated issues that CIM use has on the provision of PHC services (Hamilton, 2003; Corbin Winslow and Shapiro, 2002; Cohen *et al.*, 2005; Janamian *et al.*, 2011; Pirotta *et al.*, 2011; Poynton *et al.*, 2006; Al Shaar *et al.*, 2010; Amster *et al.*, 2000; Godin *et al.*, 2007; Ross *et al.*, 2006; Thomas *et al.*, 2003).

6.1.3 *CIM therapists in rural practice*

In addition to the impact that patient CIM use has on rural conventional PHC practice, the high utilisation and increased scope of CIM practitioners in rural areas may mean that the interface between conventional and CIM primary health care may be particularly pronounced in rural health care delivery.

For example, recent Australian research has documented the extensive role of naturopaths in providing PHC for rural communities, through the provision of culturally relevant care via treatment approaches unique to naturopathy, but also through overlapping scopes of practice with other PHC providers which are often in short supply in these areas (Wardle *et al.*, 2010).

The increased provision of PHC services by CIM providers in rural areas is also supported by the findings of a cross-sectional study of chiropractic practice in Australia, Canada and the US, which shows patients from small towns or rural areas were almost twice as likely to present with non-musculoskeletal problems as patients in urban areas (Hawk *et al.*, 2001). Smith and Carber (2002) also noted that chiropractors working in rural areas of the US had higher volume practices than their counterparts in urban areas.

One popular hypothesis for higher CIM practitioner use in rural areas is that patients are turning to CAM due to a lack of conventional PHC providers in rural areas (Featherstone *et al.*, 2003; van der Weg and Streuli, 2003; Leipert *et al.*, 2008; Trangmar and Diaz, 2008; Barish and

Snyder, 2008). This hypothesis does seem supported by some data, and a survey of rural West Texan patients, for example, found that patients who had been able to arrange an appointment for conventional care as soon as they wanted were less likely to use CIM than those patients who were not (Zhang *et al.*, 2008).

However, a CAM infrastructure audit of rural New South Wales (Australia) found that there was no inverse relationship between the numbers of conventional and CIM providers (Wardle *et al.*, 2011). Rather, lower densities of CIM providers were observed in areas with shortages of conventional providers and areas well served by conventional PHC providers were also likely to have higher numbers of CIM providers.

This finding concurs with that of a recent longitudinal analysis of 10,638 women who used CIM, which posited that access to a conventional PHC provider did not play a central role in explaining higher CIM use by women in rural and remote areas when compared with women in urban areas (Adams *et al.*, 2011). Additionally, practitioner numbers may not necessarily predict CIM utilisation, nor fully explain the higher use of CIM in rural areas. For example, Lind *et al.* (2009) found that the percentage of patients consulting a chiropractor was higher in big and small rural towns when compared with isolated regions which had the lowest availability of conventional physicians and highest comparative availability of chiropractors. Such findings highlight the need to take social and cultural factors into consideration in addition to any impact that lower access to conventional services, and increased access to CIM services, may have on rural CIM use.

6.2 Some Insights from the Field: The Perspective and Experiences of Rural GPs Regarding CIM in Rural Primary Health Care Practice

6.2.1 *Methodology*

This chapter outlines some of the insights from an emerging programme of contemporary research utilising a mixed-methods design. In order to thoroughly examine issues of practice and integration of complementary therapies in rural primary practice, qualitative interviews were employed with general practitioners practising in rural parts of the state of New South Wales, Australia. New South Wales was chosen as, in addition to being Australia's most populous state, it also has the largest rural population and most rural Divisions of General Practice of any Australian state (Australian Institute of Health and Welfare, 2010). This large rural population, combined with the geographic and demographic size and diversity of the state, provided a range of rural settings that meant findings may be more generalisable to Australia as a whole, whilst limiting data collection to one state enabled consistency in sampling and recruitment of participants.

Specifically, semi-structured, in-depth interviews were chosen for this exploratory study as they allowed for new understandings and theories to be developed during the research process and afforded an excellent means of discovering more detail about the participant's individual understandings and experiences of CAM in rural primary practice (Liamputtong and Ezzy, 2005). This format allowed participants to explain their views in detail and to highlight the most salient issues of concern to them.

The methodology for this chapter draws upon the interpretive traditions of qualitative research, focusing on establishing an in-depth understanding of the experiences of respondents. Questions were open-ended, establishing the topic or issue for discussion but not suggesting how to respond. Participants were encouraged to talk about topics in their own terms. In order to encourage natural dissemenation of opinion on behalf of the participant, the interviews did not follow a formal schedule. Throughout each interview follow-up questions were related that provided the participants an opportunity to expand, further clarify and describe their experiences and opinions as they pertained to the topic of study. Key themes, arguments and words as mentioned by the participant were noted to further probe the participant's arguments and claims at a later stage in the interview process. As far as possible, prompts were only used to ask for clarification or expansion on the participant's points.

Participants for the qualitative phase of the programme of study were drawn from respondents of an earlier survey of CIM in rural primary practice which constituted an earlier phase of this programme of research. After ethics approval was secured, all Divisions of General Practice in rural New South Wales were approached to send a 28-item questionnaire on CIM use to all GPs practising in rural New South Wales. An expression of interest to participate in the interview stage was included in the survey pack sent out to GPs. The expression of interest included a screening question, asking participants to rate their opinion of CIM on a scale of favourable to unfavourable, which was matched with survey responses to ensure that interview participants were representative of survey respondents.

The final sample in this chapter included 30 GPs who were broadly representative of Australian rural GP demographics (in regards to age, sex and length of time in practice) and practising across all degrees of rurality. Twelve respondents were female and eighteen respondents were male, which aligns with contemporary estimates that 40% of the rural GP workforce in Australia is female (Charles *et al.*, 2009), and had an average age of 53 years. Six participants were trained overseas, with training in India, South Africa, South America and the United Kingdom. This is a slight under-representative sample, as it is estimated that overseas-trained medical graduates make up 25% of Australia's medical workforce (Australian Medical Workforce Advisory Committee, 2005). The interviews lasted between 25 minutes and 92 minutes, and averaged 58 minutes.

6.2.2 *Perceptions of CIM as "alternative" and esoteric*

Andrews (2003) suggests that the therapeutic setting of some rural locations may lend themselves towards higher CIM use, with some areas being integral to the user experience of CIM due to a symbiotic relationship between CIM clinics and the local environment. Andrews utilises the example of Totnes in Devon, whose widely recognised tradition of alternative lifestyles built on spiritual awareness of the landscape complemented the development of a significant CIM industry, but acknowledges that it was a phenomenon observed in an increasing number of rural locations.

This was a notion supported in part by many participants, with several purporting that data showing higher CIM use in rural areas was tainted by the presence of outliers in pockets of "new age" and "sea-change" rural communities in rural New South Wales (such as the Northern Rivers region), rather than being reflective of what they perceived as "traditional" rural communities with agricultural, logging or mining-based economies. CIM was seen by many PHC providers as being predominantly "new-age" itself, or associated with traits related to a more cosmopolitan and affluent inner-city population, rather than aligning with conservative rural values.

This was sometimes compounded by the limited amount of CIM consumption literature that PHC providers had read which suggested that CIM users were more affluent and better educated than non-users, which was seen as being at odds with the socio-demographic profile of rural and regional Australia compared with urban populations. The lack of this new age element in many communities — as observed by the presence of health food stores, organic food stores or new age bookshops — also made PHC practitioners question the community desire for CIM services.

As such, many GPs interviewed did not believe that CIM was as important an issue in rural PHC practice as it was for their colleagues practising in urban areas. This appears related to the lack of distinction between emerging "wellness" modalities and traditional or established CIM professions by PHC providers. However, this was not the only factor affecting CIM use in rural communities; with many PHC practitioners also assuming that CIM practitioners were simply not prevalent in their rural communities, and that CIM consumption — being driven by practitioner presence — was simply not an issue in their area.

This seems to be supported in some sense in the Australian setting, with Robinson and Chesters (2008) suggesting that some forms of CIM, particularly "wellness" or "new age" modalities such as yoga, meditation and aromatherapy were more popular in "sea-change" communities as compared with traditionally agriculturally-based communities. However, the authors also observed that no such differences existed between well-established or recognised (in the Australian setting) CIM disciplines such as chiropractic or massage.

The views of GPs in rural practice conflicted with data which suggests that CIM practitioners do have a strong therapeutic footprint in rural Australia. A CIM practitioner infrastructure audit indicates that CIM practitioners make up approximately half of the PHC workforce in rural New South Wales, in both "sea-change" as well as traditionally agriculturally-based communities (Wardle *et al.*, 2011). Australian longitudinal data also suggests that rural women utilise naturopaths, herbalists and acupuncturists to the same extent as their urban counterparts (Adams *et al.*, 2007; Sibbritt *et al.*, 2007), and use some CIM practitioners — notably chiropractors and osteopaths — to a greater extent than women in urban areas (Sibbritt *et al.*, 2006). Lack of communication of CIM use by patients to their conventional PHC providers and lack of formal integrative networks between conventional and CIM practitioners may be some underlying reasons for lower prevalence of patient CIM practitioner use as perceived by rural GPs.

6.2.3 *Perceived drivers for CIM use*

When pressed, the GPs interviewed often noted that their perceptions of CIM were likely to be very different from those of their patients, with the reason for this difference usually explained in terms of patients holding "tainted" experiential views whilst GPs are able to be "objective" and develop a position based on the literature and existing evidence.

However, although most GPs had initially viewed CIM as a new-age phenomenon that may not have been directly relevant to rural patients, on reflection several respondents proffered that in some ways CIM may be attuned to the conservative nature of rural Australia.

> Medicine is always evolving, when the evidence changes we have to change too. Alternative therapies don't change and maintain their traditions. I can see how a patient would get comfort out of that, you know, getting consistent treatment for everything, particularly if every time they come to see me I have something different to say because the evidence has changed.

Other GPs also suggested that the non-subsidised nature of CIM in Australia may mean that CIM practitioners, by default, had to become more engaged and invested in their communities.

> The chiropractor here has bought a place, pumped his own money into it, and started getting to work and built up his business for 20 years. He's investing in the community, he's in Rotary. Half the GPs here probably

won't be here in five years. Their obligation for loan repayment or provider numbers or visas or whatever will end and they'll move back to the city.

Participants also thought that CIM practitioners were more likely to be originally from the area in which they practise than conventional medical providers, and as such already had cultural links and connections to the community. This concurred with previous research involving naturopathic practitioners in Australia, which suggested that the "foreign-doctor phenomenon" — whereby medical graduates from across Australia and the world were often arbitrarily pushed to practise in rural communities with little previous connection to these communities — often made it difficult to connect with rural conventional medical providers compared with CIM practitioners, particularly if their appointment was only a temporary one (Wardle *et al.*, 2010).

These cultural links were explained by the GPs as building upon other cultural aspects that encourage rural patients to seek the services of CIM practitioners over conventional providers. For example, the perception that CIM engaged the patient more in treatment than conventional medicine was felt by participants to resonate with rural values of stoicism, independence and as offering an outlet for the inventive problem-solving nature of rural patients. Additionally, it was thought that rural patients may place more emphasis on the patient–practitioner relationship and "getting their money's worth" when compared with urban patients and as such rural patients were attracted to the longer consultations that CIM practitioners were able to provide.

Rural patients' affinity for "seeing the bigger picture" was also thought to resonate with the holistic approach of CIM. This concurs with rural naturopaths' perceptions of underlying reasons for their use by rural patients (Wardle *et al.*, 2010). However, although GPs were willing to acknowledge that this may be a driver for patient use of CIM practitioners in their communities, they rejected the notion that CIM practitioners were more holistic than conventional medical practitioners practising within the biopsychosocial model of general practice, noting that naturopaths often "pushed more [natural] drugs than any medical practitioner I know" or that "chiropractors seem to treat and treat but never actually get to the underlying cause."

6.2.4 *Where to from here? A future research agenda*

Despite the recent advances in health services investigation on CIM in rural and remote communities and a growing awareness of the role CIM plays in the health care framework of rural communities, published research in this area remains minimal and there are major areas of CIM in rural PHC that require further empirical enquiry.

However, the issue of CIM has become a prevalent rural public health issue both in terms of safety and efficacy as well as in terms of the prevalence of use among rural health populations (Wardle *et al.*, 2010; Moga *et al.*, 2008). Safety issues are pronounced considering that many CIM users are by their nature vulnerable, as people often seek CIM services when they are in poorer health or conventional medicine has not been an effective strategy. Rural women in particular highlight using CIM services when they are in poor subjective health and their health needs are unmet (Williams *et al.*, 2011).

Additionally, there has been a paucity of in-depth research examining the clinical influence or impact of the CIM workforce on rural PHC. For example, although individual stakeholder perceptions have been explored, the relationship and potential interface or integration between CIM providers, patients, and conventional PHC providers in rural areas remains uncharted, as do the specific types of care CIM practitioners are providing to patients in these areas, specifically those with restricted availability of conventional PHC services.

As with many issues in rural health, CIM in rural areas is an under-researched topic. Previous exploration of this area has been minimal and this topic is only now beginning to attract detailed research attention. The existing body of work on CIM and rural health thus far has largely consisted of descriptive and cross-sectional surveys, mostly conducted in North American populations. The limited evidence available, however, seems to demonstrate that CAM use and practice in rural communities, rather than being directly related to any one push or pull factor, takes place amid a complex web of social relations and cultural networks (Wardle *et al.*, 2012).

In addition to understanding levels of CIM utilisation and integration in rural primary practice it is important to also explore and address deeper questions for which public health and health services research are particularly amenable. For example, what motivates patients in these areas to use CIM? How do populations in these areas use CIM? Are they employing CIM as a complement to conventional services or as a replacement? How do patients balance their CIM use with conventional services? If patients are using CIM instead of conventional care what has pushed them away from this care and can the factors pulling them towards CIM use be incorporated into rural PHC more generally? Are there risks associated with CIM use in rural PHC and what can be done to ameliorate them? Are there some CIM that should be more formally incorporated into rural PHC?

Issues such as those above make it difficult to identify exactly what impact and role CIM might have in the delivery of rural PHC, and what impact this has "on the ground". In order to fully comprehend the underlying drivers and influencers of CIM use in rural populations, a broader research agenda focusing on public health and health services research approaches can offer valuable insights into the interface between CIM and rural patients and practitioners, and more importantly the impact this has on PHC (Adams, 2007). These insights are essential to assist policymakers, health care planners and decision-makers, PHC providers and community planners and organisers in the face of rising CIM use in rural areas.

6.3 Conclusion

CIM appears to play an important and significant role in rural PHC. An in-depth understanding of CIM use and practice in rural health helps to provide insights for a number of health care issues which have not received substantial attention to date. These include care-seeking patterns, the realities of health care delivery, networks and provision management, as well as barriers to services in these locations. Furthermore, the prevalence of CIM use in rural communities highlights the potential volume and scope of health-seeking behaviour and activity in rural settings which have significant implications for health service management and planning, but have to date escaped empirical investigation. Further understanding of such CAM use and practice is essential in aiding the informed decision-making of rural practitioners, patients and policymakers with regards to both CAM and wider conventional care options. Such understanding serves not only to uncover how CAM affects rural primary practice, but may also help to uncover ways to make primary practice more relevant to rural communities.

References

Adams, J., Sibbritt, D., and Easthope, G. (2003). Exploring the relationship between women's health and the use of complementary and alternative medicine, *Complementary Therapies in Medicine*, **11**, 156–158.

Adams, J. (2004a). Exploring the interface between complementary and alternative medicine (CAM) and rural general practice: A call for research, *Health & Place*, **10(3)**, 285–287.

Adams J. (2004b). "Demarcating the medical/non-medical border: Occupational boundary-work within GPs' accounts of their integrative practice", in Tovey, P., Easthope, G., and Adams, J. (eds.), *The Mainstreaming of Complementary and Alternative Medicine: Studies in Social Context*, Routledge, London, pp. 140–157.

Adams, J. (2007). Restricting CAM consumption research: Denying insights for practice and policy, *Complementary Therapies in Medicine*, **15(2)**, 75–76.

Adams, J. (2008). Utilising and promoting public health and health services research in complementary and alternative medicine. The founding of NORPHCAM, *Complementary Therapies in Medicine*, **16(5)**, 245–246.

Adams, J., Sibbritt, D., Easthope, G., and Young, A. (2003). The profile of women who consult alternative health practitioners in Australia, *Medical Journal of Australia*, **179(6)**, 297–300.

Adams, J., Sibbritt, D., and Lui, C. (2011). The urban-rural divide in complementary and alternative medicine use: A longitudinal study of 10,638 women, *BMC Complementary and Alternative Medicine*, **11**, 8.

Adams, J., Sibbritt, D., and Young, A. (2007). Consultations with a naturopath or herbalist: the prevalence of use and profile of users amongst mid-aged women in Australia, *Public Health*, **121(12)**, 954–957.

Al Shaar, I., Ismail, M., Yousuf, W., and Salama, R. (2010). Knowledge, attitudes and practice of general practitioners towards complementary and alternative medicine in Doha, Qatar, *Eastern Mediterrenean Health Journal*, **16(5)**, 522–527.

Amster, M., Cogert, G., Lie, D., and Scherger, J. (2000). Attitudes and use of complementary and alternative medicine by California family physicians, *International Journal on Grey Literature*, **1(2)**, 77–81.

Andrews, G. (2003). Placing the consumption of private complementary medicine: Everyday geographies of older peoples' use, *Health & Place*, **9(4)**, 337–349.

Andrews, G.J., Adams, J., and Segrott, J. (2010). "Complementary and alternative medicine (CAM): production, consumption, research", in Brown, T., McLafferty, S., and Moon, G. (eds.), *A Companion to Health and Medical Geography*, Wiley–Blackwell, Oxford.

Andrews, G.J., Segrott, J., Lui, C., and Adams, J. (2012). "The geography of complementary and alternative medicine", in Adams, J., Andrews, G., Barnes, J., Broom, A., and Magin, P. (eds.), *Traditional, Complementary and Integrative Medicine: An International Reader*, Palgrave, Basingstoke.

Andrews, G.J., Wiles, J., and Miller, K.L. (2004). The geography of complementary medicine: Perspectives and prospects, *Complementary Therapies in Nursing and Midwifery*, **10(3)**, 175–185.

Arcury, T.A., Bell, R.A., Snively, B.M., Smith, S.L., Skelly, A.H., Wetmore, L.K., and Quandt, S.A. (2006). Complementary and alternative medicine use as health self-management: Rural older adults with diabetes, *Journals of Gerontology*, **61B(12)**, 562–570.

Australian Institute of Health and Welfare (2010). *Rural Health: The RRMA Classification,* Canberra: Australian Institute of Health and Welfare. Available at: http://www.aihw.gov.au/ruralhealth/remotenessclassifications/rrma.cfm [Accessed Nov 2011].

Australian Medical Workforce Advisory Committee (2005). *The General Practice Workforce in Australia: Supply and Requirements to 2013, AMWAC Report 2005*, AMWAC, Sydney.

Barish, R. and Snyder, A.E. (2008). Use of complementary and alternative health care practices among persons served by a remote area medical clinic, *Family and Community Health*, **31(3)**, 221–227.

Bradshaw, R., Cuff, J., Rogers, J., and Watkins, L. (2006). *Rural Disadvantage: Reviewing the Evidence*, Commission for Rural Communities, London.

Charles, J., Britt, H., and Harrison, C. (2009). "General practice workforce and workload", in Britt, H. and Miller, G. (eds.), *General practice in Australia, Health Priorities and Policies 1998 to 2008. General Practice Series No. 24*, Australian Institute of Health and Welfare, Canberra.

Cohen, M., Penman, S., Pirotta, M., and Da Costa, C. (2005). The integration of complementary therapies in Australian general practice: Results of a national survey, *Journal of Alternative and Complementary Medicine*, **11(6)**, 995–1004.

Corbin Winslow, L. and Shapiro, H. (2002). Physicians want education about complementary and alternative medicine to enhance communication with their patients, *Archives of Internal Medicine*, **162(10)**, 1176–1181.

Cueller, N., Aycock, T., Cahill, B., and Ford, J. (2003). Complementary and alternative medicine (CAM) use by African American (AA) and Caucasian American (CA) older adults in a rural setting: A descriptive, comparative study, *BMC Complementary and Alternative Medicine*, **3**, 8.

del Mundo, W.F.B., Shepard, W.C., and Marose, T.D. (2002). Use of alternative medicine by patients in a rural family practice clinic, *Family Medicine*, **34(3)**, 206–212.

Featherstone, C., Godden, D., Selvaraj, S., Emslie, M., and Took-Zozaya, M. (2003). Characteristics associated with reported CAM use in patients attending six GP practices in the Tayside and Grampian regions of Scotland: A survey, *Complementary Therapies in Medicine*, **11(3)**, 168–176.

Gesler, W.M. and Kearns, R.A. (2002). *Culture/Place/Health*, Routledge, London.

Glasgow, N., Morton, L.W., and Johnson, N.E. (eds.) (2004). *Critical Issues in Rural Health*, Blackwell Publishing, Iowa.

Godin, G., Beaulieu, D., Touchette, J., Lambert, L., and Dodin, S. (2007). Intention to encourage complementary and alternative medicine among general practitioners and medical students, *Behavioral Medicine*, **33(2)**, 67–77.

Hamilton, E. (2003). Exploring general practitioners' attitudes to homoeopathy in Dumfries and Galloway, *Homoeopathy*, **92(4)**, 190–194.

Hawk, C., Long, C., and Boulanger, K. (2001). Prevalence of nonmusculoskeletal complaints in chiropractic practice: Report from a practice-based research program, *Journal of Manipulative and Physiolological Therapeutics*, **24(3)**, 157–169.

Hoyez, A.C. (2007). The 'world of yoga': The production and reproduction of therapeutic landscapes, *Social Science and Medicine*, **65(1)**, 112–124.

Janamian, T., O'Rourke, P., Myers, S., and Eastwood, H. (2011). Information resource needs and preference of Queensland general practitioners on complementary medicines: Result of a needs assessment, *Evidence Based Complementary and Alternative Medicine*, **2011**, 810908.

Leipert, B. and Reutter, L. (2005). Developing resilience: How women maintain their health in Northern geographically isolated settings, *Qualitative Health Research*, **15(1)**, 49–65.

Leipert, B.D., Matsui, D., Wagner, J., and Rieder, M.J. (2008). Rural women and pharmacologic therapy: needs and issues in rural Canada, *Canadian Journal of Rural Medicine*, **13(4)**, 171–179.

Liamputtong, P. and Ezzy, D. (2005). *Qualitative Research Methods*, Oxford University Press, Melbourne.

Lind, B., Diehr, P., Grembowski, D., and Lafferty, W. (2009). Chiropractic use by urban and rural residents with insurance coverage, *Journal of Rural Health*, **25(3)**, 253–258.

McColl, L. (2007). The influence of bush identity on attitudes to mental health in a Queensland community, *Rural Society*, **17(2)**, 107–124.

Moga, M.M., Mowery, B., and Geib, R. (2008). Patients are more likely to use complementary medicine if it is locally available, *Rural and Remote Health*, **8**, 1028.

Ng, B., Camacho, A., Simmons, A., and Matthews, S. (2006). Ethnicity and use of alternative products in psychiatric patients, *Psychosomatics*, **47(5)**, 408–413.

Nunes, B. and Sena Esteves, M.J. (2006). Therapeutic itineraries in rural and urban areas: A Portuguese study, *Rural & Remote Health*, **6(1)**, 394.

Phelps, K. and Hassed, C. (2011). *General Practice: The Integrative Approach*, Churchill Livingstone, Sydney.

Pirotta, M., Kotsirilos, V., Brown, J., Adams, J., Morgan, T., and Williamson, M. (2011). Complementary medicine in general practice: A national survey of GP attitudes and knowledge, *Australian Family Physician*, **39(12)**, 946–950.

Poynton, L., Dowell, A., Dew, K., and Egan, T. (2006). General practitioners' attitudes towards (and use of) complementary and alternative medicine: A New Zealand nationwide survey, *New Zealand Medical Journal*, **119(1247)**, U2361.

Robinson, A. (2007). People's choice: Complementary and alternative medicine modalities, *Complementary Health Practice Review*, **12(2)**, 99–119.

Robinson, A. and Chesters, J. (2008). Rural diversity in CAM usage: The relationship between rural diversity and the use of complementary and alternative medicine modalities, *Rural Society*, **18(1)**, 64–75.

Ross, S., Simpson, C., and Mclay, J. (2006). Homoeopathic and herbal prescribing in general practice in Scotland, *British Journal of Clinical Pharmacology*, **62(6)**, 647–652.

Sherwood, P. (2000). Patterns of use of complementary health services in the South-West of Western Australia, *Australian Journal of Rural Health*, **8(4)**, 194–200.

Shreffler-Grant, J., Hill, W., Weinert, C., Nichols, E., and Ide, B. (2007). Complementary therapy and older rural women: Who uses it and who does not? *Nursing Research*, **56(1)**, 28–33.

Sibbritt, D., Adams, J., and Young, A. (2006). A profile of middle-aged women who consult a chiropractor or osteopath: Findings from a survey of 11,143 Australian women, *Journal of Manipulative and Physiological Therapeutics*, **29(5)**, 349–353.

Sibbritt, D., Adams, J., and Young, A. (2007). The characteristics of middle aged Australian women who consult acupuncturists, *Acupuncture in Medicine*, **25(1–2)**, 22–28.

Smith, M. and Carber, L. (2002). Chiropractic health care in health professional shortage areas in the United States, *American Journal of Public Health*, **92(12)**, 2001–2009.

Thomas, K., Coleman, P., and Nicholl, J. (2003). Trends in access to complementary or alternative medicines via primary care in England: 1995–2001 results from a follow-up national survey, *Family Practice*, **20(5)**, 575–577.

Trangmar, P. and Diaz, V. (2008). Investigating complementary and alternative medicine use in a Spanish-speaking Hispanic community in South Carolina, *Annals of Family Medicine*, **6**, 12–15.

van der Weg, F. and Streuli, R.A. (2003). Use of alternative medicine by patients with cancer in a rural area of Switzerland, *Swiss Medical Weekly*, **133(15–16)**, 233–240.

Wardle, J., Adams, J., and Lui, C. (2010). A qualitative study of naturopathy in rural practice: A focus upon naturopaths' experiences and perceptions of rural patients and demands for their services, *BMC Health Services Research*, **10**, 185.

Wardle, J., Adams, J., Soares-Magalhaes, R., and Sibbritt, D. (2011). The distribution of complementary and alternative medicine (CAM) providers in rural New South Wales, Australia: A step towards explaining high CAM use in rural health? *Australian Journal of Rural Health*, **19(4)**, 197–204.

Wardle, J., Lui, C., and Adams, J. (2012). Complementary and alternative medicine in rural communities: Current research and future directions, *Journal of Rural Health*, **28(1)**, 101–112.

Whorton, J. (2004). *Nature Cures: The History of Alternative Medicine in America*, Oxford University Press, New York.

Wilkinson, D., Hays, R., Strasser, R., and Worley, P. (eds.) (2004). *The Handbook of Rural Medicine in Australia*, Oxford University Press, South Melbourne.

Wilkinson, J.M. and Simpson, M.D. (2001). High use of complementary therapies in a New South Wales rural community, *Australian Journal of Rural Health*, **9(4)**, 166–171.

Williams, A., Kitchen, P., and Eby, J. (2011). Alternative health care consultations in Ontario, Canada: A geographic and socio-demographic analysis, *BMC Complementary and Alternative Medicine*, **11**, 47.

Zhang, Y., Jones, B., Ragain, M., Spalding, M., Mannschrek, D., and Young, R. (2008). Complementary and alternative medicine use among primary care patients in West Texas, *Southern Medical Journal*, **101(12)**, 1232–1237.

(Just) Who is the Expert? The Ambiguity of Expertise in Over-the-Counter CAM Purchasing: An Ethnographic Study of UK Community Pharmacies and Health Shops

Helen Cramer, Lesley Wye, Marjorie Weiss, and Ali Shaw

7.1 Introduction

Community pharmacies and health shops are examples of first-contact primary health care (PHC) as well as venues where a significant proportion of complementary and alternative medicine (CAM) products are purchased. Community pharmacies often offer a range of CAM products, and there are a small number of "integrative" pharmacists trained in both conventional and CAM. A UK survey of community pharmacists indicated that 99% sold at least one form of CAM product (including vitamin/mineral supplements) and 81% had been asked by patients/customers for a CAM product by name in the prior 12 months (Barnes and Abbott, 1999).

A significant amount of community pharmacy research has examined the pharmacist's professional role. As a profession originally concerned with the preparation of medicines, expertise in advice regarding health and illness is a more contemporary role, although it is one that has been rapidly expanding in the last 40 years (Bissell *et al.*, 2008). The role of staff in community pharmacies is more typically associated with the legal supply of prescription medicines through the 1968 Medicines Act and a focus on expert knowledge of medicines, interactions and patient safety (Hibbert *et al.*, 2002).

The recent deregulation of some prescription medicines has meant that some medicines are freely available in supermarkets, representing a challenge to both the advice-giving role of community pharmacy staff and the need to maintain profitability. In the retail environment, medicines sit on shelves next to cosmetics and a refusal of sale can lead to customers freely seeking their purchase elsewhere (Stevenson *et al.*, 2008; Hibbert *et al.*, 2002; Edmunds and Calnan, 2001).

The community pharmacy has recognised the rise of a new type of customer or consumer, one that is information-strong, information-seeking, asking critical questions, initiating dialogue and no longer necessarily accepting the authority of pharmacy staff (Traulsen and Noerreslet, 2004). Consumers are found to be increasingly confident in managing minor illnesses and conditions based on long-term personal experience (Stevenson *et al.*, 2008; Hibbert *et al.*, 2002). While some studies report that the advice of pharmacists and counter assistants is usually well received, others note that customers sometimes give strategic answers to questions in order to get what they want especially when routinised questioning styles are employed (Banks *et al.,* 2005; Hibbert *et al.*, 2002). Pharmacy staff are recognised as having expert knowledge in certain domains relevant to medications; however this expertise may not be perceived as relevant to many of the transactions, particularly those relating to CAM products (Stevenson *et al.*, 2008). Furthermore, where health advice is sought, general practitioners (GPs) are more usually seen as the key source of expertise (Bissell *et al.*, 2008; Anderson *et al.*, 2004).

Of the few research studies that have examined CAM product sales in community pharmacies, staff report frequently being asked questions about CAM products, but also report a lack of, and desire for, training (Cuzzolin and Benoni, 2009; Kwan *et al.*, 2008; Ernst, 2004; Brown *et al.*, 2008). Although potentially in an ideal position to give safety information about drug–CAM interactions (Cuzzolin and Benoni, 2009), pharmacists do not routinely document, monitor or enquire about CAM use amongst customers (Kwan *et al.*, 2008). In the rare research on sales of CAM products in health shops no information is available on training, although mystery shopping exercises have found that advice from staff in health shops is highly variable in relation to the same set of symptoms presented by the same "customer" (Reed and Trigwell, 2006).

Issues around the new consumer and the role of staff in community pharmacies and health shops relate to wider debates about the changing nature of the relationship between patients and medical professionals. A concept central to this evolving relationship is the "expert patient", which recognises that for some patients the traditional model, whereby the professional has all the knowledge and the patient accepts the decisions made on their behalf, is outdated (Charles *et al.*, 1999). Health professionals are increasingly conscious that shared decision-making or concordance with patients is desirable (Shaw and Baker, 2004; Prior, 2003; Weiss and Britten, 2003; Stevenson *et al.*, 2008). Partnership decision-making and personal responsibility for health is supported in UK health policy documents (Wilson, 2001), and patient experiences and voices are championed through government-supported health programmes (see http://www.expertpatients.co.uk/). Patients are experts in the experience of their own bodies and conditions (Prior, 2003). Health information is increasingly available and accessible, especially on the Internet with medical science increasingly under scrutiny (Fox *et al.*, 2005; Hibbert *et al.*, 2002; Wilson, 2001). These developments facilitate patient access to information and increase patient involvement in decisions about their health.

Critics of the expert patient model point out that it falsely places patient experience on an equal footing with medical training and education (Fox and Ward, 2006; Stevenson *et al.*, 2008). It is argued that patients cannot diagnose (Prior, 2003), that structural constraints and entrenched professional power is underestimated (attributable to Tang and Anderson 1999 in Fox and Ward, 2006), and that professionals do not value patients' beliefs, often block patients' decisions and try to control information (Fox and Ward, 2006). Some researchers argue that while some patients may adopt a more active and informed role others may not possess the necessary competencies or wish to take responsibility for their health (Flyn *et al.*, 2006; Fox *et al.*, 2005; Stevenson *et al.*, 2008). Lupton (1997) argues that when people are sick, in pain or afraid they are less likely to pursue treatments and decisions as rational and independent consumers but might prefer to place their faith and trust in health professionals (also Cornish and Gillespie, 2009). Lupton (1997) also argues that it is this dependency when feeling sick or ill that is the major barrier to consumerism rather than patients being any less knowledgeable than professionals.

CAM customers are thought more likely to constitute the "new consumer" (Sharma, 2003). They may be like expert patients and be information rich, fully shouldering the responsibility for their own health and purchasing products on the advice of a CAM practitioner or have the experience of successfully managing a chronic condition. The asymmetry of knowledge and training between professionals and customer may not be as great when buying CAM over-the-counter, especially because we know that CAM training is lacking. On the other hand, some CAM customers may be turning to CAM in desperation having exhausted all conventional biomedical treatments and, like Lupton (1997) suggests, be seeking staff and wanting advice in which to place their faith. They may alternatively be thoroughly confused by an overload of health information which is perhaps even harder to evaluate given the contested nature of CAM scientific evidence (Lambert, 2006; Ernst, 2004).

CAM products available in health shops and community pharmacies represent a multitude of different philosophies of health, illness and approaches to healing. Given this diversity it would be surprising if staff were knowledgeable about all the products associated with those divergent philosophies. There is also variability in staff training and seniority in a shop where a pharmacist might have a very different level of knowledge and training compared with a pharmacy counter assistant. Allowing for the huge range of CAM products, associated philosophies, training opportunities and health conditions, perhaps customers are greater experts on a given health condition or CAM product than pharmacy and health store staff? The study reported in this chapter examines the selling and purchase of CAM products over-the-counter in community pharmacies and health shops from the perspective of relative expertise. When it comes to buying over-the-counter CAM products just *who* is the expert: customers, shop staff or medical practitioners?

7.2 Subjects and Methods

7.2.1 *Study design and definitions*

An ethnographic approach including semi-structured interviews and non-participant observation was selected to provide in-depth examination of the everyday work and roles of pharmacy and health shop staff, detailed observation of interactions between staff and customers and flexibility and triangulation to compare what is said with what is done (Silverman, 2001). For the purposes of this study the definition of CAM products included: homeopathic products, anthroposophical remedies, flower remedies, herbs, food supplements (e.g., spirulina, aloe vera, probiotics, enzymes) and single vitamins and minerals (e.g., vitamin C, zinc). We excluded: multivitamins, antenatal vitamins, body building products and weight loss products.

7.2.2 *Sampling and data collection*

Purposeful sampling was used to identify a range of "information rich" settings selling CAM products (Patton, 2002). These included "mainstream" pharmacies where CAM products were a relatively marginal part of the business, "integrated" pharmacies that had a strong focus on CAM products alongside conventional treatments, and health shops that focused entirely on CAM products. The final sample included three pharmacies and three health shops, both chain stores and independent retailers. Whilst maintaining maximum variation, it was possible to choose six very different settings in one UK city located within half a mile of each other. As all the shops in the sample were geographically close, customers could therefore potentially choose which setting to shop in.

Twenty-four staff team members (including pharmacists, owners/managers and counter assistants) across the six settings were interviewed face-to-face. Thirty customers were selected across the settings and approached to participate in subsequent telephone interviews following observation of a CAM-related interaction with staff. Customers were selected to maximise variation in terms of age, gender, types of CAM product purchased and nature of interaction with staff (e.g., advice seeking or purchase only).

Observations in each setting were undertaken over a one month period and were conducted at different times of the day and over the weekend to ensure that a range of customers were represented. A total of 107 hours were spent observing across all six settings and included observation of 97 CAM-related purchases and instances of advice giving. Some interactions did not involve a purchase and some involved the purchase of more than one product. The volume of CAM-related purchases and customer-staff interactions in the six settings varied considerably.

7.2.3 Data analysis

The interviews were recorded and transcribed for analysis. Data analysis was largely thematic and guided by the principles of the constant comparative method (Strauss and Corbin, 1998). The observations were recorded using handwritten notes which were written up into more detailed notes shortly following the close of the observation period and then transcribed for analysis.

We developed codes, initially drawing on the topic guides and then increasingly in response to themes emerging from the data. The analysis of the observation data was supplemented and triangulated by data from the staff and customer interviews.

7.3 Findings

After introducing the basic differences between the six study sites, we will compare the claims of expertise from customers, health shop staff and pharmacy staff that were found in each of the six settings. We first examine the views (and behaviour) of customers buying the CAM products and include the products bought, the health issues to be addressed and the stage in the help-seeking pathway where CAM products were bought over-the-counter. The chapter then focuses upon the claims to expertise of those selling CAM products including focus upon the training staff received, the resources at their disposal and the protocols and safeguards to which staff referred.

7.3.1 Comparison and description of study sites

The key characteristics of each of the six study sites is given in Table 7.1.

As shown in Table 7.1, the study sites varied significantly in terms of products (other than CAM). The reported proportion of CAM sales as a total of overall sales in most settings (actual or estimated by pharmacists/managers), ranged from 5% to 66%. The sports health shop, chain

Table 7.1 Key characteristics of each of the six study sites.

Study site	Chain or independent?	Own brands?	What else sold in shop	CAM sales*
Independent health shop	Independent	No	Health foods, cosmetics, books, environmental products	22%
Clinic health shop	Chain	Yes	Cosmetics, books	15%
Sports health shop	Chain	Yes	Health foods, sports supplements	66%**
Homeopathic pharmacy	Independent	No	Toiletries, some health foods	30%
Independent pharmacy	Independent	No	Toiletries, stationary	5%
Chain pharmacy	Chain	Yes	Toiletries, cosmetics, food	6–7%

* Proportion of CAM sales represented as a total of overall sales in shop — actual or estimate.
** Likely to be over-representation as includes sports supplements not considered CAM in this study.

pharmacy and clinic health shop were all part of a chain that sold own-brand products and had selling targets for staff. The most competitive prices for CAM products were in the sports health shop and chain pharmacy, with the latter having a permanent three for two offer on all CAM products and vitamins.

7.3.2 *Health conditions and most commonly bought products*

The health issues for which customers bought CAM products ranged from the minor and acute to the chronic and serious. Half of the over-the-counter CAM product purchases were for symptomatic or curative purposes, a quarter of the purchases were for preventative reasons and it was not possible to say the purpose of the final quarter. The most common curative reasons for which people were buying CAM included: coughs and colds (e.g., herbs such as mallow and elderflower), bruising/surgical recovery (homeopathic arnica) or sleep problems (e.g., homeopathic coffea and herbal valerian). The products bought for preventative reasons included those used as constitutional remedies, as tonics or immunity boosts (e.g., homeopathic cuprum ferrum and Echinacea), for diet supplementation (e.g., vitamin B12 for vegans and extra iron for breastfeeding mothers), for preventing certain health problems such as colds (e.g., vitamin C, Echinacea), cystitis (golden seal), migraines (homeopathic bidor and rhus tox) and digestive problems (silium), and to counteract the possible side effects of taking allopathic products (e.g., protobiotics for antibiotics and the enzyme Co-Q-10 for customers taking statins).

Overall, of the 97 observations, the most common purchases were: herbs (32), food supplements (23), single vitamins or minerals (18), homeopathic or anthroposophical medicines or homeopathic/herbal mixtures (18) and essential oils (6). Loose herbs were regularly bought in combination, e.g., colt's foot and skull cap which partly explains why herbs are the most common observed purchase.

7.3.3 Customer help-seeking pathway and information sources

Some customers viewed over-the-counter CAM products as the most appropriate first port of call. Treatments for use at home were sometimes bought for curative purposes, sometimes desired for preventing worsening of health issues or to prevent anticipated future health problems. For example, one customer bought homeopathic apis to restock her home remedies and said she usually cared for her family members with CAM before any visits to the doctor:

> I try self-treat at home first … I grew up in the States and medicine, medical care is very expensive there. And also my grandfather had been a doctor and well, I suppose partly because of cost and partly because we found it worked, we started with homeopathy or whatever else, and then if that didn't work we went to the doctor (Customer A, homeopathic pharmacy).

Other customers purchased over-the-counter CAM as a last resort, often having already sought advice from other sources including doctors or CAM therapists. Whether or not a customer used CAM products as a first choice or a last choice appeared related to their confidence, experience and satisfaction of using CAM. For example, a woman, aged 40, bought valerian tincture for her son's sleep problems, and arnica and manuka honey for her mother who was about to have an operation. She said:

> My eldest son, when he had a very serious operation when he was very lit-tle, and I used arnica then, and it was very successful … my eldest son has Asperger's syndrome so sleeping is very, very difficult indeed … so we're doing everything we can to just try and relax him … it was two of [sons' name]'s school friends who actually told me about it. They said that you can get it in tea … and so that's why we tried it … being a mother who has a child who's got Asperger's syndrome, you feel, well, when you're first told it, because I had never heard of it before, I was very upset … [after diagnosis] I just proceeded to read book after book after book … it's nice that people can spend time with you and explain things to you … you feel you've gone from one extreme, knowing nothing at all and you just, you want to absorb as much information to help your child in every possible way that you can (Customer B, independent health shop).

Our analysis identifies customers as using a wide variety of sources of information and help-seeking routes prior to CAM purchases. Some cus-tomers drew upon advice from family or friends and some had previously seen a CAM practitioner. A few customers were collecting (homeopathic) prescriptions on the advice of a holistic GP, while others had read books, magazines or newspaper articles, had used the Internet, and/or had experi-mented with other CAM products previously. For example, one woman aged 49 was observed collecting a prescription for homeopathic Ferrum Quartz from the homeopathic pharmacy. In an interview afterwards, she listed the CAM products that she took (evening primrose oil, omega 3 and 6, Echinacea, cranberry tablets, devils claw, vitamin C), the conventional drugs (amytriptyline, propranolol and Imigran) and the practitioners she consulted (private nutritionist) for her problems with headaches, migraines and chronic fatigue syndrome:

> People are trying to be more health conscious I think and healthy and I think that's why they try so many things… well, a bit like me. I mean, I,

I have no evidence to, to suggest that evening primrose helps me at all or cod liver oil. You just read what you read and then think well, why not? It might help so, yeah (Customer C, homeopathic pharmacy).

Some customers reported working closely with their GP, especially in those cases where the GP was also a holistic practitioner. For example, a German woman, aged 52, described a relationship with doctors from her holistic GP surgery as well as a private London specialist doctor for her chronic conditions (rheumatoid arthritis and Sjorgrens syndrome). This woman was observed in the homeopathic pharmacy collecting a prescription for homeopathic antiomonite for shingles which she said she had correctly self-diagnosed. Her diagnosis was then confirmed by her GP whose prescription addressed the "crabby" feelings she had. She said that she took a conventional joints drug and high doses of vitamin D on the recommendation of her specialist doctor and did the Alexander Technique. She had also sought advice and CAM products previously from the independent health shop for restless leg syndrome, as well as buying CAM on the Internet.

Other customers reported that for certain health problems they no longer asked their GPs advice but stuck to what worked. For example a woman, aged 31, was observed buying homeopathic belladonna for her son who had just had a course of antibiotics for an ear infection which had made his eczema worse. Through a variety of experiences this woman implies that she might be consulting her doctor less in the future:

He's had it [eczema] since he was born… I didn't know where else to go, so I started seeing a homeopath and basically, to cut a long story short, I've been seeing her for about seven months and his skin's like brilliant, it's like really nice… He'd tried pretty much everything that he could for his, you know, his age… some of the creams are so strong and his skin was awful… he was like a little cornflake… he had this ear infection, I took him to the doctor, they've given him antibiotics and basically what it's done, it's sent him back say, two months' worth of working on his skin… and I'd rather not do that again, so I've got the belladonna here, ready for if he's got another infection, I can give him that instead of going to the doctor… [My doctor] referred me to a dermatologist and when I went to see him and I said to him, you know, I did ask him straight out, I said "do you believe

in homeopaths?" and he said "no I don't", he said "they're absolute
rubbish"… I do believe in [homeopathy], I really do, because he's [son]
completely different, because his behaviour was so naughty as well… and
I really don't understand it at all [laughter] but, it works for [son's name]
so that's good enough for me (Customer D, independent pharmacy).

The types of advice-seeking observed also reveal where customers were
situated in the help-seeking pathway (see also Cramer *et al.*, 2009). For
example, one third of the 97 customers observed had a diagnosis for their
problem but wanted help to find some sort of remedy. Another third of
customers had a prior diagnosis and a general idea of a remedy that would
be suitable, but wanted help from staff as to which specific product to purchase. This need for help in choosing amongst the range of available products is not surprising given that, for example, the sports health shop sold
11 different types of evening primrose oil and 16 different types of B vitamins. A number of customers needed help with diagnosis but all were
advised to seek a diagnosis elsewhere. The longest discussions and most
complex advice-seeking were observed in the independent health shop,
clinic health shop and homeopathic pharmacy. There was some evidence
that customers were deliberately choosing certain shops when they wanted
more complex advice and would then seek less expensive high street retail
options or the Internet once they had identified the products required.

7.3.4 *Evidence of customers as experts and non-experts*

A number of customers buying CAM over-the-counter were experts in
some way. Some customers were experts on their own conditions through
the reading they had done or the bodily knowledge they had from products
they had tried and their previous routes for advice. One example is a man,
aged 47, who bought colloidal silver for his wife's eye infection after first
trying advice from the chain pharmacy and eye hospital. The man said that
he had consulted a herbalist on occasion but mostly self-medicated and
read widely about CAM and nutrition:

I think there is some research for colloidal silver but you would not necessarily say it's worked. It's never specific, it's like the colds and the flu,

vitamin C seems to help… we went to the eye hospital. They said there was no treatment for a virus infection… [also] used eye baths of Optrax [*sic*] or something, she went to [chain pharmacy] last week and talked to the pharmacist there. We tried these but told not to bother at the eye hospital they said chemical eye treatments would make it worse so don't use them, they said, you can't do much just wait for it to clear up, no treatment… It's [CAM] a hobby, I've always been interested in it, perhaps it's a neurotic hobby. I should have been a doctor, I enjoy it, I enjoy the self-medication approach. … I just like experimenting and experiencing (Customer E, sports health shop).

Some customers described a type of expertise that relied on the support of a CAM practitioner. For example, one man, aged 40, bought quassia chips for head lice on the advice of his children's teacher. In an interview afterwards his wife said that the whole family regularly consulted a homeopath and that she herself was trained in reflexology. She said that she did use conventional drugs for her blood pressure as well as seeing a kinesiologist and acupuncturist. She reported having experimented with CAM products and indicated an awareness of her limitations as an expert:

This last pregnancy and birth I was really quite poorly with pre-eclampsia and stuff, so I'm having blood pressure pills and stuff like that so we do use it when it's necessary… and I think self-prescribing can be a danger as well … I once proved a remedy I was trying on my husband for asthma and I made him a lot worse and that was my lesson… So I discussed it immediately with my homeopath and she told me not to do that again (Customer G, clinic health shop).

The customers described or displayed what could be termed "expertise" in a number of different ways: through their bodily knowledge of having tried products, through having tried conventional allopathic approaches, through reading up on their condition, through consultations with practitioners trained in CAM or sometimes from their own CAM training. In addition, four customers reported in interviews that they were trained allopathic doctors. For example, one woman, who was training as an eye surgeon, was buying arnica in the chain pharmacy because her senior colleague recommended it to all his patients.

7.3.5 *Staff knowledge, training and experience regarding CAM products*

An overall assessment of the level of knowledge of staff in the six study sites can be separated into the following components: background training in alternative therapies, length of experience in an advisory role, specific knowledge about products, and the resources and support in order to follow up any queries, see Table 7.2.

As shown in Table 7.2 the six study sites varied enormously with respect to training and experience; staff in the clinic health shop, the independent health shop and homeopathic pharmacist appeared to be better trained regarding CAM products compared with staff in the other three sites. Furthermore, the routes through which staff across the sites gained their experience and training varied widely. For example, trained acupuncturists and homeopaths in the clinic health shop seemed to have a depth of knowledge of a specific CAM discipline acquired through their professional training, whereas the detailed product-based knowledge of staff in the independent health shop had been acquired through more everyday "learning on the job" over a number of years. In contrast, at the sites where staff had more superficial knowledge, summary information about CAM products appeared to be learned by rote for fortnightly knowledge tests conducted by managers.

In two of the three pharmacies there was a clear disparity between the pharmacists' level of knowledge and commitment to CAM and the scepticism of most counter assistants interviewed. The following quote illustrates this point:

> But are you really looking after the health of that patient, or are you just fobbing them off... with homeopathic, you know, you're finding what the problem is and trying to get that problem out of the body and making that person into a better person, a normal person, rather than suppressed really, you know, that's the issue with sort of allopathics, ... on antidepressants ... you're suppressing them to a certain level (Pharmacist E, homeopathic pharmacy).

Pharmacy and counter assistants in the chain pharmacy stood out as the least trained and knowledgeable about CAM products. With very limited

Table 7.2 Comparison of key characteristics of the six study sites.

Study site	Staff training, length of experience in role and resources used
Independent health shop	Staff have diplomas in health food retail, attend short courses on CAM, receive training from company representatives and do their own "research". Several have many years' experience in an advisory role. Use manufacturers' hotlines extensively. A CAM/pharmaceutical interactions database is available for customer use.
Clinic health shop	One qualified CAM practitioner is present among the staff at all times. Staff attend an induction course. Mostly younger staff with few years' experience in role. Staff use CAM reference books extensively. Company researcher contact. Other hotlines and databases not used.
Sports health shop	Staff attend short induction and advanced courses. Have fortnightly product training and testing. No hotlines used and few CAM reference books. Company product information is main CAM reference source.
Homeopathic pharmacy	Pharmacist is training to be a qualified homeopath. Counter assistants attend company representative courses and a six-month correspondence CAM course. Several have many years' experience in advisory role. Use hotlines regularly, as well as CAM reference books and CAM/pharmaceutical interactions database.
Independent pharmacy	One of the two pharmacists has completed a six-month homeopathy course and own reading. Counter assistants have no CAM training. Some CAM reference books used and hotlines. Customer CAM database that did not work.
Chain pharmacy	Pharmacists have fortnightly allopathic product updates including some CAM products. Counter assistants have no CAM training. One CAM reference book and no hotlines used.

training in CAM, both pharmacists in interviews explained that they only felt comfortable recommending CAM remedies of which they had personal experience.

All the shops had established selling protocols which highlighted significant differences in the selling styles of the health shops and pharmacies. For example, staff in the sports health shop were observed to regularly ask about medication use but routinely sent their customers next door to the big chain pharmacists to check on any medications and inter-actions. In the clinic health shop the staff in-house protocol emphasised empowerment and responsibility.

Staff in two of the pharmacies used a variation of the WWHAM protocol (who for, what symptoms, how long had it, allergies, any other medication?) for CAM products as for allopathic ones. With especially poor knowledge about CAM products in the chain pharmacy even the importance of following a protocol was not fully understood by all staff members, as is shown by the following interview extract:

> R: If it's herbal stuff off the shop floor, not really, I just look at the back of the packet and just… I don't know, we don't really WWHAM them.
> I: So you don't really ask: "How long have you had it for? What other medications are you using?"
> R: Not on herbal stuff no. From our point of view, because we haven't had the training, we just presume it's like vitamins… basically we would just scan them through the till. Normally with paracetamol it will ask us to prompt them. It will prompt us just to check to see if they have used it before… whereas if it's herbal stuff, there's no actual prompt on the till for us to actu-ally follow a WWHAM protocol for herbal stuff… it would just go through as a 3 for 2 offer on vitamins (Counter Assistant G, chain pharmacy).

7.3.6 *Expertise and non-expertise amongst staff*

The variable training with regards to CAM products of staff in pharmacies and health shops illustrates that CAM expertise is not always guaranteed in these settings. Indeed, in a field as large as CAM which embraces such a diverse range of therapeutic philosophies and traditions, it would be unrealistic for staff to be sufficiently trained in all areas. Expertise around products is to be distinguished from expertise of a more in-depth knowledge of a CAM approach. In some instances, the radical alternative views of health care and healing exemplified by some staff stood out and represented in-depth CAM expertise and knowledge:

> Most chronic disease is caused by nutritional deficiency or an environmental situation and you cannot address either of those with drugs. If you're suffering from a lack of vitamin C no amount of aspirin is going to correct

that situation… you know, if you take a non-steroidal, the first thing you've got to do is repay the damage it's done to your gut every time. Every time you take an aspirin your stomach bleeds, and it's not just the stomach, but what's the structure, what's happening to the structure of the stomach as a result of that. How much damage is being done, what resources do you have to repair it? Most people haven't, so they end up with a leaky gut that leads to candida and all kinds of things. Call it the drug cascade effect… we get so many people coming into the shop who are absolutely distressed because they've got to take all of this iron because the doctor's recommended it, and it's making them so sick and the doctor just says, well tough. And we give them things which are alternatives and they go away and they just are amazed, (i) because the dose, they have to take a lower dose, and (ii) because it works much faster. And they think it's a miracle, and there's nothing miraculous about it, it's just that doctors… well basically doctors are not trained in nutrition and they have a mindset that says, well nutrition can't be important because if it were important we'd be trained in it. We're not trained in it, therefore it can't be important. And therefore they ignore and have almost a blind spot… all they know is drugs, they have no other concept (Manager I, independent health shop).

7.4 Discussion

The central question underlying this chapter has been "who is the expert?", when customers buy CAM products over-the-counter in health shops and community pharmacies. The findings of this study have shown that staff training in CAM was highly variable as were the resources they could draw upon although there were several examples of very good training and resources. There was some evidence of "new consumers", information rich and information-seeking customers, asking critical questions (Traulsen and Noerreslet, 2004). These knowledgeable customers often had extensive experience of a condition and the available treatments and sometimes reported the advice of a number of other experts such as CAM practitioners or (holistic) GPs. A significant proportion of customers sought advice on products and treatment approaches and therefore sought expertise from community pharmacy and health shop staff. Although some customers were just purchasing products and knew exactly what they wanted, others needed and sought in-depth advice. These findings are therefore not consistent with the study of Stevenson *et al.* (2008) set in community pharmacies where staff advice was irrelevant to customers. Consistent with previous research on CAM (Bissell *et al.*, 2008; Anderson *et al.*, 2004; Adams, 2000), GPs were still a cornerstone of people's health management even when they were rarely the main source of advice for CAM purchases (with the exception of holistic GP practices).

There was evidence of customers experimenting with CAM products which has also been noted by other researchers (Nichter and Thompson, 2006; Doel and Segrott, 2003). This is perhaps partly due to CAM approaches which facilitate and encourage positive health and assumptions that CAM products are safe as has also been found in other studies (Ben-Arye *et al.,* 2008). This evidence of experimentation lends support to the idea of CAM customers as new consumers, experts of their own bodies, confident and responsible for their own health and embracing the status of expert patient. The expert patient model emphasises that patients are experts by virtue of their experiences but also of their embodiment (Pedersen and Baarts, 2010). It is also possible from our study to distinguish different styles of expertise between health shop staff and pharmacy staff via the use of protocols and store physical environment, pharmacy staff seemed to favour a paternalistic approach to health advice giving in contrast to health shop staff, who tended to advise via a partnership approach.

7.5 Conclusion

The position and role of the expert is more open to negotiation between staff and customers in over-the-counter CAM purchasing situations. The relative expertise in a situation depends on the degree and quality of advice previously sought by a customer, the type of health condition experienced, their experience of previous treatments, previous bodily experiences and whether the products are curative or preventative in their purpose and aim. Some customers gained expert status through their experiences, their bodies and accumulated knowledge. Some staff had expert knowledge of conditions and products via training and experience and appeared to recommend appropriate products at least in terms of customer needs. However, not all customers were clear about their requirements and likewise not all staff were trained in CAM and there was evidence that suggested these staff members would not be able to advise suitable CAM products. The over-the-counter relationship between customers and staff, with regards to CAM purchases, had differences to the more frequently theorised patient–health professional relationship, although this remains a useful model. For example, CAM users could perhaps be considered at one end of the spectrum of professional–patient relationships, as "consumers" who are particularly proactive, self-helping and information seeking. This is either because conventional medicine has failed them, or because they have a "healthy consumer" philosophy that embraces the use of whatever works to maintain health and well-being. As an under-researched area of first contact primary care, this study has examined the ambiguity of expertise in over-the-counter CAM purchases. Given the prevalence of CAM purchases and information seeking, it appears important for staff and professionals in these PHC settings to obtain further CAM training and expertise. There is reason to be optimistic regarding such a development given the many examples of good quality training and expertise identified in this study upon which further advances can build.

Acknowledgements

Special thanks to all the staff in health shops and community pharmacies that took part in this study and the customers who spoke to us about their purchases. We would also like to thank and acknowledge our funders, the Avon Primary Care Research Collaborative.

References

Adams, J. (2000). General practitioners, complementary therapies and evidence-based medicine: The defence of clinical autonomy, *Complementary Therapies in Medicine*, **8(4)**, 248–252.

Anderson, C., Blenkinsop, A., and Armstrong, M. (2004). Feedback from community pharmacy users on the contribution of community pharmacy to improving the public's health: A systematic review of the peer reviewed and non-peer-reviewed literature 1990–2002, *Health Expectations*, **7**, 191–202.

Banks, J., Shaw, A., and Weiss, M. (2005). Walking a line between health care and sales: The role of the medicines counter assistant, *The Pharmaceutical Journal*, **274**, 586–589.

Banks, J., Shaw, A., and Weiss, M. (2007). The community pharmacy and discursive complexity: A qualitative study of interaction between counter assistants and customers, *Health and Social Care in the Community*, **15(4)**, 313–321.

Barnes, J. and Abbott, N.C. (1999) Experiences with complementary remedies: A survey of community pharmacists, *The Pharmaceutical Journal*, **263(7063)**, 114–118.

Ben-Arye, E., Frenkel, M., Klein, A., and Scharf, M. (2008). Attitudes toward integration of complementary and alternative medicine in primary care: Perspectives of patients, physicians and complementary practitioners, *Patient Education and Counseling*, **70(3)**, 395–402.

Bissell, P., Blenkinsop, A., Short, D., and Mason, L. (2008). Patients' experiences of a community pharmacy-led management service, *Health and Social Care in the Community*, **16(4)**, 363–369.

Bissell, P., Ward, P.R., and Noyce, P.R. (1997a). Variation within community pharmacy — 1. Responding to requests for over-the-counter medicines, *Journal of Social and Administrative Pharmacy*, **14**, 1–15.

Bissell, P., Ward, P.R., and Noyce, P.R. (1997b). Variation within community pharmacy — 2. Responding to the presentation of symptoms, *Journal of Social and Administrative Pharmacy*, **14**, 105–115.

Brown, J., Morgan, T., Adams, J., Grunseit, A., Toms, M., Roufogolis, B., Kotsirilos, V., Pirotta, M., and Williamson, M. (2008). *Complementary Medicines Use and Needs of Health Professionals: General Practitioners and Pharmacists*, NPS, Australia.

Charles, C., Gafni, A., and Whelan, T. (1999). Decision-making in the physician–patient encounter: Revisiting the shared treatment decision-making model, *Social Science & Medicine*, **49(5)**, 651–661.

Collyer, F. (2004). "The corporatisation and commercialisation of CAM", in Tovey, P., Easthope, G., and Adams, J. (eds.), *The Mainstreaming of*

Complementary and Alternative Medicine: Studies in Social Context, Routledge, London.

Cornish, F. and Gillespie, A. (2009). A pragmatist approach to the problem of knowledge in health psychology, *Journal of Health Psychology*, **4(6)**, 800–809.

Cramer, H., Shaw, A., Wye, L., and Weiss, M. (2009). Over-the-counter advice seeking about complementary and alternative medicines (CAM) in community pharmacies and health shops: An ethnographic study, *Health and Social Care in the Community*, **18(1)**, 41–50.

Cuzzolin, L. and Benoni, G. (2009). Attitudes and knowledge toward natural products safety in the pharmacy setting: An Italian study, *Phytotherapy Research*, **23(7)**, 1018–1023.

Doel, M.A. and Segrott, J. (2003). Beyond belief? Consumer culture, complementary medicine and the disease of everyday life, *Environment and Planning D: Society and Space*, **21**, 739–749.

Edmunds, J. and Calnan, M.W. (2001). The reprofessionalisation of community pharmacy? An exploration of attitudes to extended roles for community pharmacists amongst pharmacists and general practitioners in the United Kingdom, *Social Science & Medicine*, **53(7)**, 943–955.

Ernst, E. (2004). Complementary medicine pharmacist? *The Pharmaceutical Journal*, **273**, 197–198.

Flyn, K.E., Smith, M.A., and Vannes, D. (2006). A typology of preferences for participation in healthcare decision-making, *Social Science & Medicine*, **63**, 1158–1169.

Fox, N. and Ward, K. (2006). Health identities: From expert patient to resisting consumer, *Health*, **10(4)**, 61–479.

Fox, N., Ward, K., and O'Rourke, A.J. (2005). The "expert patient": Empowerment or medical dominance? The case of weight loss, pharmaceutical drugs and the Internet, *Social Science & Medicine*, **60**, 1299–1309.

Hassell, K., Harris, J., Rogers, A., Noyce, P., and Wilkinson, J. (1996). *The Role and Contribution of Pharmacy in Primary Care*, National Primary Care Research and Development Centre, Manchester.

Hibbert D., Bissell, P., and Ward, P.R. (2002). Consumerism and professional work in the community pharmacy, *Sociology of Health & Illness*, **24(1)**, 46–65.

Kwan, D., Boon, H.S., Hirschkorn, K., Welsh, S., Jurgens, T., Eccott, L., Heschuk, S., Griener, G.G., and Cohen-Kohler, J.C. (2008). Exploring consumer and pharmacist views on the professional role of the pharmacist with respect to natural health products: A study of focus groups, *BMC Complementary and Alternative Medicine*, **8**, 40.

Lambert, H. (2006). Accounting for EBM: Notions of evidence in medicine, *Social Science & Medicine,* **62(11)**, 2633–2645.

Lupton, D. (1997). Consumerism, reflexivity and the medical encounter, *Social Science & Medicine*, **45(30)**, 373–381.

Nichter, M. and Thompson, J.J. (2006). For my wellness, not just my illness: North Americans' use of dietary supplements, *Culture, Medicine & Psychiatry*, **30**, 175–222.

Patton, M.Q. (2002). *Qualitative Research and Evaluation Methods*, Sage, London.

Pedersen, I.K. and Baarts, C. (2010). "Fantastic hands" — But no evidence: The construction of expertise by users of CAM, *Social Science & Medicine*, **71(30)**, 1068–1075.

Prior, L. (2003). Belief, knowledge and expertise: The emergence of the lay expert in medical sociology, *Sociology of Health and Illness*, **25**, 41–57.

Reed, J.E. and Trigwell, P. (2006). Treatment recommended by health shops for symptoms of depression, *Psychiatric Bulletin*, **30**, 365–368.

Reid, S. (2002). A survey of the use of over-the-counter homeopathic medicines purchased in health stores in central Manchester, *Homeopathy*, **91(4)**, 225–229.

Sharma, U. (2003). "Medical pluralism and the future of CAM", in Kelner, K., Wellman, B., Pescosolido, B., and Saks, M. (eds.), *Complementary and Alternative Medicine: Challenge and Change*, Harwood Academic Publishers, Amsterdam.

Shaw, J. and Baker, M. (2004). "Expert patient" — dream or nightmare? *British Medical Journal*, **328**, 723–724.

Silverman, D. (2001). *Interpreting Qualitative Data: Methods for Analysing Talk, Text and Interaction*, Sage, London.

Stevenson, F.A., Leontowitsch, G., and Duggan, C. (2008). Over-the-counter medicines: Professional expertise and consumer discourses, *Sociology of Health and Illness*, **30(6)**, 913–928.

Strauss, A.L. and Corbin, J. (1998) *Basics of Qualitative Research: Grounded Theory Procedures and Techniques*, Sage, London.

Thomas, K.J., Nicholl, J.P., and Coleman, P. (2001). Use and expenditure on complementary medicine in England: A population based survey, *Complementary Therapies in Medicine*, **9(1)**, 2–11.

Thompson, T. and Feder, G. (2005). Complementary therapies and the NHS, *British Medical Journal*, **331**, 856–857.

Traulsen, J.M. and Noerreslet, M. (2004). The new consumer of medicine: The pharmacy technicians' perspective, *Pharmacy World & Science*, **26**, 203–207.

Vincent, C. and Furnham A. (1996). Why do patients turn to complementary medicine? An empirical study, *British Journal of Clinical Psychology*, **35(1)**, 37–48.

Weiss, M. and Britten, N. (2003). What is concordance? *The Pharmaceutical Journal*, **271**, 493.

Willis, E. and White, K. (2004). "Evidence based medicine", in Tovey, P., Easthope, G., and Adams, J. (eds.), *The Mainstreaming of Complementary and Alternative Medicine*, Routledge, London.

Wilson, P.M. (2001). A policy analysis of the expert patient in the United Kingdom: Self-care as an expression of pastoral power? *Health and Social Care in the Community*, **9(3)**, 130–142.

Part Three

Conceptualising Integrative Medicine in Primary Health Care: Experience and Challenges

Integrating Complementary Medicine in Primary Health Care as a Response to Contemporary Challenges: A Focus upon Effectiveness Gaps and Self-Care

David Peters

In this chapter I identify three distinct yet interrelated crises facing contemporary primary health care: cost (and cure), care, and commitment (and compassion), and explore the possibility of complementary medicine (CM) providing a possible means to address these problems. I argue that self-care and complementary and alternative medicine (CAM) remain a challenge for doctors despite being crucial to the ability of contemporary medicine to engage effectively with patients with long-term conditions. I also explore how self-care and CM may support doctors' engagement with the art of medicine.

8.1 CM in Primary Health Care: Signpost or Destination?

The sustained popularity of CM over recent decades may be partly interpreted as reflecting patients' perception and experiences of conventional medicine and/or doctors. While diverse in detail, most CM shares a certain orientation — an ecology of ideas that sets them apart from radical reductionist biomedicine (Coulter, 2004). CM's intellectual territory is in many ways the opposite of what biomedicine has become: perhaps most obviously by not separating mind from body nor health problems from personal predicaments. At a time when radical forms of biomedicine are implicitly impersonal and sometimes explicitly dehumanising, CM at its best is — in theory at least — biopsychosocial (as indeed, conventional medicine at its best still can be). Furthermore, CM resonates with aspirations for health care that is personal and small-scale rather than general and industrialised, accepts the subjectivity of illness as well as objective signs of disease, perceives social and emotional predicaments as significant, aims to provide meaning and encourage self-healing, fosters engagement, participation and co-creation on behalf of the patient and employs "natural" materials and methods wherever appropriate.

It is worth noting at this point that most of these characteristics can be incorporated into mainstream medicine. Biomedicine is well positioned to respond to disease, and biomedical technologies excel when acutely ill patients need to be passive recipients of high-tech treatment. Even though we celebrate this, medicine in its more technological modes is less well equipped for collaborating with the body's self-healing processes, or for making peace in the body-mind. Therefore, in managing long-term conditions where the therapeutic alliance, engagement and self-care — aspects of the art of medicine — must come to the fore, it will be far less effective.

8.2 CM and UK General Practitioners

In primary health care, where clear causes and distinct cures are generally less obvious than in hospital medicine, the realities of biopsychosocial holism are hard to ignore. Here, general practitioners (GPs) witness every day how people's health swings in the balance between resilience and vulnerability. Yet we still know too little about the ways the biological, the psychological and the social interact. Bearing these uncertainties, many of the UK's GPs have nonetheless suggested to their patients that they try CM (Thomas et al., 2001). Qualitative research also reveals the depths of support for CM amongst UK GPs (Adams, 2000; 2001a; 2001b; 2003; 2004; Adams and Tovey, 2000).

Despite the fact some doctors may have become more sceptical about CM in recent years, and even though many local NHS organisations have cut their spending on CM, its popularity with patients seems not to have waned. One explanation for the continuing popularity of CM (even in the face of opposition from a range of commentators), may be that these medicines still signify public and professional aspirations for more gentle and humane forms of health care. The popularity of CM amongst doctors partly lies in the ability of CM to help address areas of practice where conventional medicine has faced major challenges — in particular, chronic illness and stress-related and painful conditions. Most CM clients have previously received conventional medical treatment, and surveys show high levels of satisfaction with their experience of CM, and useful outcomes (Sharples *et al.*, 2003; Ernst and White, 2000).

The gradual integration of CM into the NHS mainstream indicates a growing acceptance of CM, an acceptance paralleled by an emergent public awareness on the one hand of health risks and lifestyle, and on the other of environmentalism; along with the collapse of deference to experts, a distrust of technological fixes, and a wish to avoid becoming dependent on either. Astin (1998), drawing upon US research, suggests that "...along with being more educated and reporting poorer health status, the majority of alternative medicine users appear to be doing so not so much as a result of being dissatisfied with conventional medicine but largely because they find these health care alternatives to be more congruent with their own values, beliefs, and philosophical orientations toward health and life" (Astin, 1998, p. 1550). GPs swim in the same cultural pool as their patients, so seen against this backdrop we could interpret the popularity of CM as linked to resurgent concerns about resilience and sustainability. We ought not to disregard, however, the genuine absence of low-cost, "natural", safe alternatives to drugs for many common primary health care problems whose pharmaceutical treatments may be ineffective or unacceptable to patients. These "effectiveness gaps" (Fisher *et al.*, 2004) are why some GPs use or recommend CM. As for the evidence base, though there may be some relevant randomised clinical trials (RCTs), evidence is more likely to be from GPs' own clinical impressions and patient anecdotes (Peters *et al.*, 2001). The possible parallels between CM use and improved self-care might further encourage some primary care commissioners, struggling to maintain an NHS already threatened by underfunding, to consider CM as a cost-saving exercise.

8.3 Integrating CM into Mainstream Primary Health Care

Why might doctors working in family practice take the trouble to engage with or even practise CM? Conventional medicine has had a limited impact on the pandemic chronic diseases of industrial societies. Stress-mediated, environment-mediated and lifestyle-mediated disease, addiction and psychological disorders seem to respond partially if at all. Nor does the biomedical model easily cope with "undifferentiated disease", the ordinary "unwellness" that affects all of us some of the time. Not surprisingly it is in primary health care, where people manage their own health problems or seek advice from a wide range of professionals, that CM is making its presence most keenly felt (Adams, 2004; Adams and Tovey, 2000).

GPs' clinical time is mostly spent dealing with acute self-limiting diseases which get better on their own, with chronic or terminal structural disease, and with long-term relapsing disorders, such as asthma or skin problems — dysfunctional conditions, often with a significant "stress-related" component. Patients' problems with daily living and their social crises also occupy a significant amount of GPs' time. Struggling to meet this range of needs, GPs more readily than hospital specialists, would agree that health care is only partly a matter of science, and that biomedicine has no "cure" for many of the problems patients bring to them (Adams, 2000). This has led to curiosity in CM amongst many doctors and their patients about providing effective (and less potentially harmful) treatments and a practical way of enhancing self-healing processes (Adams, 2003).

Primary health care involves both "doing to" and "being with" patients, and the "doing to" aspects of practice are in transition. The boom in anti-depressant prescribing and the advent of poly-pharmacy for cardiovascular disease and diabetes management have ushered in a "biologised" style of primary care, so that a great deal of GP time (and generating income) is now taken up with meeting centrally defined standard operating procedures. As a consequence, the "being with" aspects of GP work and the doctor–patient relationship are changing and, for those GPs who feel the pull of more timeless notions of health and healing, the attraction of CM systems is obvious: their expansive respect for subjective lived-experience, illness-narrative and the body as a whole, balances biomedicine's focus on cells and tissues, diagnostic symptoms and objective signs.

Perhaps then CM, rather than being a destination in itself, is a signpost and a way of reconstructing the clinical transaction, and a flag of allegiance to a less reductionistic world view. Astin's (1998) conclusion that having a holistic philosophy of health is predictive of alternative health care use, probably applies to doctors as well as their patients. If so, patients sensing certain practitioners' allegiance to this world view would find their approach and advice more in tune with their own health beliefs than biomedicine's drier offerings. In some instances this congruence, along with time and touch, and the intention to integrate rather than reduce and fragment, will induce non-specific effects which evoke changes not only in the minds of patients, but in their bodies too (Benedetti *et al.*, 2005). Powerful context-bound "meaning responses" (Moerman and Jonas, 2002), plus advice about lifestyle and support for positive change are part and parcel of CM therapies at their best. All these "human factors" can be brought to bear in conventional care too, and with good effect. However, GPs are currently preoccupied with Quality Outcomes Frameworks aimed at preventing chronic disease through evidence-based scientific management. Whatever CM's strengths with chronic illness and distress, it is not effective in severe acute or life-threatening disease, and biomedicine can often relieve or palliate where CM alone would fail. Integrative medicine in primary health care can draw on the entire spectrum.

Integrative medicine must marry the science with the art of medicine and, in various ways, CM has highlighted these challenges and perhaps signposted possible solutions. It has made us more curious about the limitations of experimental studies, the controversy of efficacy versus effectiveness, and reawakened interest in the therapeutic relationship and the mysterious placebo response. At a time when emerging technologies demonstrate the futility of our old notions of mind and body as separate, CM claims that it attends to the lived-body and the "whole person". Like narrative medicine, CM is concerned about individual predicaments, about resilience or its lack, about the context in which illness arises and how people and relationships adapt. CM also generally insists that people must engage in some form of self-care. At this most critical time for bio-medicine, these are crucial messages.

8.4 Crisis? What Crisis?

Biomedicine's technological advances against disease have paid dividends but not without costs: soaring budgets, side effects, resistant infections and, for many patients, a dependence upon daily medication use over extensive periods. While lip service is paid to primary health prevention and the crucial role of primary health care for population health, the hospital sector still consumes the lion's share of resources.

How can contemporary health care find its way out of these binds? Where, if anywhere, does CM fit into this? Crises of cure and cost are two sides of the same coin, but medicine is faced with deeper crises. With its time-honoured place in society changing rapidly, medicine appears to be losing the authority and respect it once attracted; and at the same time a mechanistic vision of health care is threatening its once unquestioned benevolent values. If these two trends are connected, then no amount of new magic bullets or bolted-on CM will address the underlying existential crises of compassion and commitment which biomedicine currently faces. In contrast, the arts of caring are losing ground arguably because until quite recently their softer story could not be told in the hard language of cell biology. In fact biomedicine's tacit assumption that people are individual, separate biochemical machines serves to diminish our sense of a shared humanity. All this (along with sheer overwork) could explain why many doctors and nurses say they are unhappy in health care (Smith, 2012).

8.5 Sustainable Primary Health Care?

In the last two decades NHS costs have climbed from below 5% to more than 8% of the gross domestic product (GDP). In England, life expectancy for men increased by about five years, but healthy life expectancy by less than three. This means that more people are old and sick — mainly due to chronic mental and physical illness (White, 2010). Obesity already affects one in four people in England, and the associated health care costs are estimated to be £3.7 billion a year, rising to £6.3 billion within four years. It is estimated that one in four people in England will experience at least one significant mental health issue at some point in their life. The consequences cost the country £105 billion a year in health and social care services and lost economic output (NHS, 2012). Pharmaceutical solutions alone will not get to the root of problems such as these.

When considered alongside the World Health Organization's all-embracing yardstick of health as a state of *complete* physical, mental and social well-being (and not merely the absence of disease or infirmity) most of us are, and will ever remain, unhealthy. As for the absence of disease, new screening technologies will soon mean there are no normal patients, only those who have not yet been sufficiently investigated. And, if the pharmaceutical industry keeps naming new "diseases", and intervention thresholds for lowering cholesterol, blood pressure and glucose continue to fall, the already dwindling ranks of the physically and psychologically healthy will shrink still further. As for infirmity, given that living longer with one or more long-term diseases is now the later-life norm, "complete health" is sure to have eluded most of the half a million people who die each year in England, two thirds of whom are over 75 years old — let alone the 17% of the present UK population predicted to live to 100 years (Department of Work and Pensions, 2010).

This prediction, of course, is largely dependent on the assumption that such widespread life-extension is desirable, and achievable by the same means that has already stretched life expectancy among the more affluent in the UK to over 85 years. To the extent that these extra years are either given to us, or supported by the NHS, we should expect the life expectancy curve to flatten out as NHS resources effectively shrink year-on-year. For, as deficit-reduction curtailment begins to bite, inevitably, services we have taken for granted will disappear. Faced with longer waiting lists and overstretched, patchy services we will have to find more efficient ways of delivering health care. Staff costs represent 60% of the NHS budget, so a diminished workforce seems likely, but this would only work if NHS users were prepared to engage far more with their own care and improved lifestyles. Are patients going to be willing to do more for themselves? And if they are, will health professionals know how best to support them?

Any GP who has attempted to change patients' help-seeking behaviour knows it is not easy. As GPs we all have patients with common minor health problems, who keep returning to us even though our relatively ineffective prescribing has done no more than punctuate years of disappointing consultations that leave us and our patients dissatisfied. Arguably we foster their dependency every time we prescribe in this way. Yet most GPs would agree that self-care/self-management is crucial in long-term conditions and that in chronic relapsing "effectiveness gaps" such as irritable bowel syndrome (IBS), mild to moderate depression and back pain, lifestyle, relaxation skills and exercise can make or break recovery. Other effectiveness gaps include primary dysmenorrhea, perimenopausal problems, persistent fatigue, "fibromyalgia", tension-type headaches, migraine, poor sleep and undifferentiated illness related to "stress". What is more, many patients who have a chronic diseases such as diabetes, ischaemic heart disease, chronic congestive heart failure and chronic obstructive pulmonary disease, also have the same sorts of ill-defined, hard to treat symptoms. In many cases they undermine life quality more than the primary condition itself, provoke repeated GP visits, fruitless investigation and frustrating hospital referrals.

8.6 CM and Self-care: A Note about "Effectiveness Gaps"

Although in the current climate doctors are urged to implement evidence-based medicine, "effectiveness gap" events are relatively common. The validity of this term is supported by a survey of 22 London-based family doctors which highlighted a total of 78 clinical problems representing 57 clinical areas subject to effectiveness gaps (Fisher *et al.*, 2004). Since almost half of these clinical problems occurred more than once a week and the rest between one and four times a month, effectiveness gaps appear to be a significant clinical problem in everyday primary health care.

The most frequently identified areas for effectiveness gaps are musculoskeletal problems, including osteoarthritis, inflammatory arthritis, back pain and soft tissue syndromes. Depression was the second most frequently cited clinical area. Others were eczema, chronic pain (excluding back pain), IBS, headache and rhinitis. Lack of efficacy was the most common reason given, but unacceptability of treatment to patients and poor compliance (possibly linked to adverse effects) were also important.

The UK's Self-Care Campaign Group reported that "of the 57 million consultations which involved a minor ailment, 51.4 million are for minor ailments alone; a testament to an NHS addressing demand rather than need" (Self-Care Campaign Group, 2010). It would appear that we need to start learning about, talking about and supporting self-care, not only for the sake of our patients and in order that clinicians can take better care of their own health, but also for the very survival of the NHS. This is going to call for a change of attitude among patients and health care practitioners alike.

Well-informed self-care could be an under-tapped resource with immense potential to improve the health and well-being of people suffering from long-term conditions, and which might reduce their dependency on prescribed medication. Better supported self-care — which could include aspects of CM — would help control runaway health care costs and make our industrialised health care systems more cost-effective even as costs soar and ever-aging populations make heavier demands. Tackling the culture of dependency within medicine is a challenge requiring attention. By doing so, GPs who inform, support and signpost self-care options effectively will be able to boost patients' resilience, reduce their reliance on medication and prevent relapses.

Interestingly, the use of CM is very high among people with long-term conditions, and most of it is "self-care" in as much as it is not provided by the NHS, and patients choose and pay for it themselves; care not directed by a health professional, or if it is, by one whom the patient has chosen, rather than by their GP. Researchers at the Peninsula School of Medicine and Dentistry (MacKichan *et al.*, 2011) surveyed 3,000 people on GP lists and found that self-care (including self-paid CM) was already widespread for common problems such as back pain, fatigue, stress problems, headache and menopause problems, particularly among those most bothered by their symptoms. Common self-care approaches identified in this research also included medicinal products (nutritional, homeopathic, herbal, etc.), dietary change, psychological techniques, and complementary therapies provided by non-NHS practitioners including acupuncture, manual therapies and a variety of others as well as classes and mind-body methods such as yoga, meditation and t'ai chi.

This research also found that for the primary health care patients surveyed, doctors and health professionals were the most trusted sources of advice, though friends and relatives also had a powerful influence on their decision-making about self-care. Yet those who do use CM often do not discuss this with their doctors. Perhaps because they suspect GPs will be uninformed about CM or unsympathetic to these approaches (Owen *et al.*, 2001). Indeed, GPs report knowing little about CM, would like to learn more, and would be more favourably disposed towards CM if shown a convincing evidence base (Milden and Stokols, 2004). However, there has been no single evidence-based, easy-to-use source of self-care information for patients or their GPs, which takes account of a wide range of lifestyle, mind-body and CM options with reliable links to research evidence supporting their use. Consequently, when patients discuss self-care or CM with their GPs, these options may not be systematically explored or well supported with easily accessed written material.

Recognising this gap and supported by the UK Department of Health, researchers at the University of Westminster searched for the available evidence for self-care in 12 typical "effectiveness gaps". These are: back pain, sore muscles (fibromyalgia), tiredness and fatigue, sleep problems, feeling low and depression, stress and anxiety, headache, migraine, IBS, osteoarthritis, period problems and hot flushes.

The information gathered is now available at an interactive website (http://selfcare-library.info/). The site explains each condition, indicates when to seek medical advice, and rates the options (exercise, relaxation, diet, over-the-counter medicines, supplements and natural remedies, classes and therapies) for likely benefit, safety and cost. Included on the website are PDFs about each condition and users, should they wish, can click through to abstracts of all the papers cited, on screen and so (perhaps in conversation with their practitioner) make better-informed choices. The content is too extensive to summarise in this chapter but readers can easily view the site and its references online. Tables 8.1 and 8.2 at the end of this chapter provide an example of how the Self-Care Library works.

Mild-moderate depression is arguably one of conventional medicine's "effectiveness gaps". The example given is intended to illustrate how self-care (with or without CM) might broaden GPs' evidence-based options for managing clinical challenges such as these.

8.7 The Impact of CM: Beyond the Quick Fix

Self-care and CM can help doctors deal more effectively with long-term conditions. However, this is not because CM provides "magic bullets" and quick fixes. It would be a mistake to see CM options as purely technical; as reified commodities that can be separated from the person who provides them. Consequently, an acupuncture treatment or an osteopathy session is quite unlike a course of antibiotics. Even so, drugs are much more effective with certain patients and in some contexts than others. So it requires a well-designed RCT to weed out the individual differences, biases and "therapeutic relationship", and other "non-specific effects", in order to reveal the technical efficacy of the drug itself. Hence the RCT serves only to show whether, on average, in whosoever hands, an intervention will be of use to the population as a whole (so far, so generalisable). However, individual transactions in CM are not like this — a practitioner's skills and a range of individual patient characteristics are all part and parcel of what determines treatment outcomes. The technical, manual, intellectual, emotional and communicative abilities of a practitioner cannot be generalised, nor can patients' differing capacities for making sense, engaging in change or triggering self-regulating processes. At this practitioner–patient interface the art of medicine becomes entirely relevant, even though scientific biomedicine tends to marginalise this category of knowledge.

Conventional pharmaceuticals undeniably have an important role in the management of chronic illness and disease: but the notion that a chronic or relapsing health problem can be "fixed" is arguably counterproductive. Rather than raising inappropriate expectations of cure, a more realistic aim is the co-production of health: and here, the therapeutic focus needs to shift towards concern for resilience, well-being, maintenance of function and containment of distress. The "self-care CM orientation" can help reconfigure the therapeutic task, and re-engage the art of medicine.

8.8 Conclusions

The assumption that medicine can solve all human problems and that it will in time find ways of curing all diseases, has resulted in the over application of the biomedical paradigm. The costs for "delivering" this system of care have become too great to be sustained and, despite this vast expenditure, users all too often complain that they feel fragmented and disempowered. This raises the question of whether medicine's intense emphasis on technology, and the public sector's drive to industrialise health care "delivery" in the name of equity and efficiency, has undermined traditional values of service and compassion, and its respect for healing processes. CM's popularity could be a warning that the "biologisation" of medicine is undermining other, time-honoured humanistic dimensions. There are widespread intimations that too many practitioners now find their work stressful and alienating.

Self-care names a broad area of endeavour with roots in public health, whereby communities and individuals prevent disease, promote health and manage their own illnesses through informed choices and organised efforts. Self-care is now of urgent concern for society as a whole and for all organisations, both public and private (Wanless, 2002). Though the case for self-care is very strong, medical education and attitudes, practice and funding give it too little attention. Sustainability, well-being and resilience are emerging cultural watchwords, and allegiance to holistic world views have been linked to patients' use of CM, whose growing popularity has been paralleled by a burgeoning interest in self-care and healthier lifestyles. It has been proposed that doctors may find a "self-care complementary medicine" orientation to be of value not only practically, but also as a way of enacting a holistic perspective which helps them cope better with many kinds of health problems that do not fit easily into the biomedical paradigm.

Research into why doctors engage with CM could help us better understand medicine's "effectiveness gaps", and address deficiencies in the humanistic dimensions of medical education and practice. CM and self-care are "complex interventions" and the question of whether their use in primary health care actually promotes self-regulation in chronic illness and disease will involve pragmatic and naturalistic methods as well as the experimental. Emerging psychophysiological research models are already revealing insights into self-healing processes and mechanisms of co-regulation. This new knowledge will in time change the way we think about medicine, treat disease and promote health.

Translating the self-care/CM orientation into practice calls for a pluralistic primary health care team; some senior doctors have already found this way of working to be personally and clinically valuable. Clearly, this reorientation can only prove cost-effective in the long-term, but it would be a mistake to underestimate the potential added value of re-embracing self-care and CM — the sustainability of health care professionals and the organisations they work in may depend on marrying medical science with the art of medicine. The need to restore the service ethic to medicine and to embed compassion and holism at the core of medical practice are now priority issues and there is emerging empirical evidence to suggest the union of self-care and CM within primary health care could be one possible means of addressing some of the contemporary challenges facing this core area of health care provision.

Table 8.1 How the Self-Care Library codes the evidence, safety and cost.

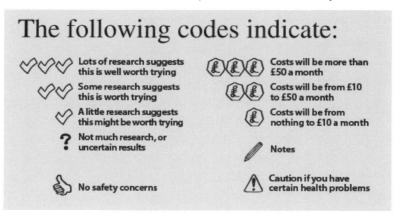

The following codes indicate:

- ✓✓✓ Lots of research suggests this is well worth trying
- ✓✓ Some research suggests this is worth trying
- ✓ A little research suggests this might be worth trying
- ? Not much research, or uncertain results
- 👍 No safety concerns
- 💷💷💷 Costs will be more than £50 a month
- 💷💷 Costs will be from £10 to £50 a month
- 💷 Costs will be from nothing to £10 a month
- ✏ Notes
- ⚠ Caution if you have certain health problems

Table 8.2 An example of the way the Self-Care Library categorises information.

| | | | Mild-moderate depression | |
	Evidence	Safety	Cost	Evidence
Changes to lifestyle				
Books and audio	✓✓	☜	£–££	**Self-help interventions for depressive disorders and depressive symptoms: A systematic review.** Morgan, A.J. and Jorm, A.F. (2008). *Annals of General Psychiatry,* **7**,13. **Self-help books for depression: How can practitioners and patients make the right choice?** Anderson, L., Lewis, G., Araya, R., Elgie, R., Harrison, G., Proudfoot, J., Schmidt, U., Sharp, D., Weightman, A., and Williams, C. (2005). *British Journal of General Practice,* **55**, 387–392.
Creative distraction	✓✓	☜	£	**Self-help interventions for depressive disorders and depressive symptoms: A systematic review.** Morgan, A.J. and Jorm, A.F. (2008). *Annals of General Psychiatry,* **7**,13.
Exercise	✓✓	☜	£	**Self-help interventions for depressive disorders and depressive symptoms: A systematic review.** Morgan, A.J. and Jorm, A.F. (2008). *Annals of General Psychiatry,* **7**,13. **A Countryside for Health and Well-Being: The Physical and Mental Health Benefits of Green Exercise.**

(*Continued*)

Table 8.2 (*Continued*)

	Mild-moderate depression			
	Evidence	Safety	Cost	Evidence
				Pretty, J., Griffin, M., Peacock, J., Hine, R., Sellens, M., and South, N. (2005). *Report for the Countryside Recreation Network.* Available at: http://www.essex.ac.uk/ces/occasionalpapers/Kerry/CRN%20Report%20FINAL%20Feb14.pdf [Accessed Nov 2011] **Exercise for depression.** Mead, G.E., Morley, W., Campbell, P., Greig, C.A., McMurdo, M., Lawlor, and D.A. (2009). *Cochrane Database of Systematic Reviews,* Issue 3. Art. No.: CD004366. DOI: 0.1002/14651858.CD004366.pub4.
Relaxation techniques	✓✓	☞	£	**Relaxation for depression.** Jorm, A.F., Morgan, A.J., and Hetrick, S.E. (2008). *Cochrane Database of Systematic Reviews,* Issue 4. Art. No.: CD007142. DOI: 10.1002/14651858.CD007142.pub2.
Self-help on the Internet	✓	⚠	£	**Self-help interventions for depressive disorders and depressive symptoms: A systematic review.** Morgan, A.J. and Jorm, A.F. (2008). *Annals of General Psychiatry,* **7**,13. **Internet-based cognitive behaviour therapy for symptoms of depression and anxiety: A meta-analysis.** Spek, V., Cuijpers, P., Nyklicek, I., Riper, H., Keyzer, J., and Pop, V. (2007). *Psychological Medicine,* **37**, 319–328. **Status of computerised cognitive behavioural therapy for adults.** Titov, N. (2007). *Australian and New Zealand Journal of Psychiatry,* **41**, 95–114.

(*Continued*)

Table 8.2 *(Continued)*

			Mild-moderate depression
	Evidence	Safety	Cost	Evidence
Special diets	?	☞	£	**Self-help interventions for depressive disorders and depressive symptoms: A systematic review.** Morgan, A.J. and Jorm, A.F. (2008). *Annals of General Psychiatry*, **7**,13. Potential for helpful longer-term effects was found for autogenic training, light therapy, omega-3 fatty acids, pets and prayer. Many of the trials were poor quality and may not generalise to self-help without professional guidance. **BluePages Depression Information.** The Centre for Mental Health Research, The Australian National University. Available at: http://bluepages.anu.edu.au/.
Buy something over-the-counter (OTC)				
Herbals				
St John's wort				
Nutritional supplements				
Omega 3	✓	⚠	£–££	**A meta-analytic review of double-blind, placebo-controlled trials of antidepressant efficacy of omega-3 fatty acids.** Lin, P.Y. and Su, K.P. (2007). *Journal of Clinical Psychiatry*, **68**(7),1056–1061. **Effects of n-3 long-chain polyunsaturated fatty acids on depressed mood: Systematic review of published trials.**

(Continued)

Table 8.2 (*Continued*)

Mild-moderate depression

	Evidence	Safety	Cost	Evidence
				Appleton, K.M., Hayward, R.C., Gunnell, D., Peters, T.J., Rogers, P.J., Kessler, D., and Ness, A.R. (2006). *American Journal of Clinical Nutrition*, **84(6)**,1308–1316.
				Do essential fatty acids have a role in the treatment of depression? Williams A.L., Katz D., Ali A., Girard, C., Goodman, J., and Bell, I. (2006). *Journal of Affective Disorders*, **93(1–3)**,117–123.
				Cross-national comparisons of seafood consumption and rates of bipolar disorders. Noaghiul, S. and Hibbeln, J.R. (2003). *American Journal of Psychiatry*, **160**, 2222.
SAMe	✓✓	⚠	££	**Self-help interventions for depressive disorders and depressive symptoms: A systematic review.** Morgan, A.J. and Jorm, A.F. (2008). *Annals of General Psychiatry*, **7**,13.
Vitamins	✓	⚠	£	**Folate, vitamin B12, homocysteine, and the MTHFR 677CT polymorphism in anxiety and depression: The hordaland homocysteine study.** Bjelland, I., Tell, G., Vollset, S., Refsum, H., and Ueland, P. (2003). *Archives of General Psychiatry*, **60**, 618–626.
				Serum 25-hydroxyvitamin D and depressive symptoms in older women and men. Milaneschi, Y., Shardell, M., Corsi, A.M., Vazzana, R., Bandinelli, S., Guralnik, and Ferrucci, J.M. (2010). *Journal of Clinical Endocrinology & Metabolism*, **95(7)**, 3225–3233.

(*Continued*)

Table 8.2 (*Continued*)

			Mild-moderate depression
	Evidence	Safety	Cost	Evidence
				Effects of vitamin D supplementation on symptoms of depression in overweight and obese subjects: Randomised double blind trial.
				Jorde, R., Sneve, M., Figenschau, Y., and Svartberg, J. (2008). *Journal of Internal Medicine*, **264**(**6**), 599–609.
				Vitamin D and mood disorders among women: An integrative review.
				Murphy, P. and Wagner, C. (2008). *Journal of Midwifery & Women's Health*, **53**(**5**), 440–446.
				Self-help interventions for depressive disorders and depressive symptoms: A systematic review.
				Morgan, A.J. and Jorm, A.F. (2008). *Annals of General Psychiatry*, **7**,13.
				Folate for depressive disorders.
				Taylor, M.J., Carney, S.M., Geddes, J., and Goodwin, G. (2003). *Cochrane Database of Systematic Review*, Issue 2. Art. No.: CD003390. DOI: 10.1002/14651858.CD003390
Light box	✓	⚠	£££	**Light room therapy effective in mild forms of seasonal affective disorder: A randomised controlled study.**
	✓			Rastad, C., Ulfberg, J., and Lindberg, P. (2008). *Journal of Affective Disorders*, **108**(**3**), 291–296. Epub 28 Nov 2007.
				Short exposure to light treatment improves depression scores in patients with seasonal affective disorder: A brief report.
				Virk, G, Reeves, G., Rosenthal, N.E., Sher, L., and Postolache, T.T. (2009). *International Journal on Disability and Human Development*, **8**(**3**), 283–286.

(*Continued*)

Table 8.2 (*Continued*)

			Mild-moderate depression	
	Evidence	Safety	Cost	Evidence
				Self-help interventions for depressive disorders and depressive symptoms: A systematic review. Morgan, A.J. and Jorm, A.F. (2008). *Annals of General Psychiatry*, **7**,13.
				Light therapy for non-seasonal depression. Tuunainen, A., Kripke, D.F., and Endo, T. (2004). *Cochrane Database of Systematic Reviews*, Issue 2. Art. No.: CD004050. DOI: 10.1002/14651858.CD004050.pub2.
Practitioners or classes				
Acupuncture	?	☞	££-£££	**Acupuncture for depression.** Smith, C.A., Hay, P.P.J., and MacPherson, H. (2010). *Cochrane Database of Systematic Reviews*, Issue 1. Art. No.: CD004046. DOI: 10.1002/14651858.CD004046.pub3.
Autogenic training	✓	☞	££	**Autogenic training: A meta-analysis of clinical outcome studies.** Stetter, F. and Kupper, S. (2002). *Applied Psychophysiology and Biofeedback*, **27(1)**, 45–98.
				Self-help interventions for depressive disorders and depressive symptoms: A systematic review. Morgan, A.J. and Jorm, A.F. (2008). *Annals of General Psychiatry*, **7**,13.

(*Continued*)

Table 8.2 (*Continued*)

Mild-moderate depression

	Evidence	Safety	Cost	Evidence
Exercise programmes	✓✓✓	👉	£	**Exercise for depression.** Mead, G.E., Morley, W., Campbell, P., Greig, C.A., McMurdo, M., and Lawlor, D.A. (2009). *Cochrane Database of Systematic Reviews*, Issue 3. Art. No.: CD004366. DOI: 10.1002/14651858.CD004366.pub4. **Self-help interventions for depressive disorders and depressive symptoms: A systematic review.** Morgan, A.J. and Jorm A.F. (2008). *Annals of General Psychiatry*, **7**,13.
Homeopathy	?	👉	££	**Homeopathy for depression: A systematic review of the research evidence.** Pilkington, K., Kirkwood, G., Rampes, H., Fisher, P., and Richardson, J. (2005). *Homeopathy*, **94(3)**, 153–163.
Massage	✓	👉	££	**Massage therapy for the treatment of depression: A systematic review.** Coelho, H.F., Boddy, K., and Ernst, E. (2008). *International Journal of Clinical Practice*, **62(2)**, 325–333. **A meta-analysis of massage therapy research.** Moyer, C.A., Rounds, J., and Hannum, J.W. (2004). *Psychological Bulletin*, **130(1)**, 3–18. **A meta-analysis of massage therapy research.** Moyer, C.A., Rounds, J., and Hannum, J.W. (2004). *Psychological Bulletin*, **130(1)**, 3–18.

(*Continued*)

Table 8.2 *(Continued)*

Mild-moderate depression

	Evidence	Safety	Cost	Evidence
Psychological therapies	✓✓✓	☞	££	**Aromatherapy and massage for depression: A systematic review.** Pilkington, K., Kirkwood, G., Rampes, H., and Richardson, J. (2006). *Complementary and Alternative Medicine Evidence Online (CAMEOL) Database.* **Psychotherapy for depression.** Hermann, E.K., Munsch, S., Biedert, E., and Lang, W. (2010). *Therapeutische Umschau,* **67(11)**, 581–584.
Yoga	✓	☞	£-££	**Yoga for depression: The research evidence.** Pilkington, K., Kirkwood, G., Rampes, H., and Richardson, J. (2005). *Journal of Affective Disorders,* **89(1–3)**,13–24. SR of 5 RCTs. **Self-help interventions for depressive disorders and depressive symptoms: A systematic review.** Morgan, A.J. and Jorm, A.F. (2008). *Annals of General Psychiatry,* **7**, 13.

References

Adams, J. (2000). General practitioners, complementary therapies and evidence-based medicine: The defense of clinical autonomy, *Complementary Therapies in Medicine*, **8(4)**, 248–252.

Adams, J. (2001a). Enhancing holism? General practitioners' explanations of their complementary practice, *Complementary Health Practice Review*, **6(3)**, 193–204.

Adams, J. (2001b). Direct integrative practice, time constraints and reactive strategy: An examination of general practioner therapists' perceptions of their complementary medicine, *Journal of Management in Medicine*, **15(4)**, 312–322.

Adams, J. (2003). The positive gains of integration: A qualitative study of general practitioner therapists' views of their complementary practice, *Primary Health Care Research and Development*, **4(2)**, 158–167.

Adams, J. (2004). "Demarcating the medical/non-medical border: Occupational boundary-work within GPs' accounts of their integrative practice", in Tovey, P., Easthope, G., and Adams, J. (eds.), *The Mainstreaming of Complementary and Alternative Medicine: Studies in Social Context*, Routledge, London, pp. 140–157.

Adams, J. and Tovey, P. (2000). "Complementary medicine and primary care: Towards a grass-roots focus", in Tovey, P. (ed.), *Contemporary Primary Care: The Challenges of Change*, Open University Press, Buckingham, pp. 167–182.

Astin, J.A. (1998). Why patients use alternative medicine. Results of a national study, *Journal of the American Medical Association*, **279(19)**, 1548–1553.

Benedetti, F., Mayberg, H.S., Wager, T.D., Stohler, C.S., and Zubieta J. (2005). Neurobiological mechanisms of the placebo effect, *The Journal of Neuroscience*, **25(45)**, 10390–10402.

Coulter, I. (2004). "Integration and paradigm clash: The practical difficulties of integrative medicine", in Tovey, P., Easthope, G., and Adams, J. (eds.), *The Mainstreaming of Complementary and Alternative Medicine: Studies in Social Context*, Routledge, London, pp. 103–119.

Evans, J. (2011). Number of future centenarians by age group, April 2011, Department of Work and Pensions. Available at: http://statistics.dwp.gov.uk/asd/asd1/adhoc_analysis/2011/centenarians_by_age_groups.pdf [Accessed June 2012].

Ernst, E. and White, A. (2000). The BBC survey of complementary medicine use in the UK, *Complementary Therapies in Medicine*, **8(1)**, 32–36.

Fisher, P., Van Haselen, R., Hardy, K., Berkovitz, S., and McCarney, R. (2004). Effectiveness gaps: A new concept for evaluating health service and research needs applied to complementary and alternative medicine, *Journal of Alternative and Complementary Medicine*, **10(4)**, 627–632.

MacKichan, F., Paterson, C., Henley, W., and Britten, N. (2011). Self-care in people with long term health problems: A community based survey, *BMC Family Practice*, **12**, 5.

Milden, S.P. and Stokols, D. (2004). Physicians' attitudes and practices regarding complementary and alternative medicine, *Behavioral Medicine*, **30(2)**, 73–82.

Moerman, D.E. and Jonas, W.B. (2002). Deconstructing the placebo effect and finding the meaning response, *Annals of Internal Medicine*, **136**, 471–476.

NHS. (2012). Mental health services, Available at: http://www.nhs.uk/NHSEngland/AboutNHSservices/mentalhealthservices/Pages/Overview.aspx [Accessed Sept 2012].

Owen, D., Lewith, G.T., and Stephens, C.R. (2001). Can doctors respond to patients' increasing interest in complementary and alternative medicine? *British Medical Journal*, **322**, 154–157.

Peters, D., Chaitow, L., Morrison, L., and Harris, G. (2001). *Integrating Complementary Therapies in Primary Care*, Harcourt Brace, Edinburgh.

Sharples, F.M., Van Haselen, R, and Fisher, P. (2003). NHS patients' perspective on complementary medicine: A survey, *Complement Therapies in Medicine*, **11(4)**, 243–248.

Smith, R. (2012). British nurses 'burnt-out' study finds, *The Telegraph*, 22 Mar. Available at: http://www.telegraph.co.uk/health/healthnews/9158427/British-nurses-burnt-out-study-finds.html [Accessed Mar 2012].

The Self-care Campaign Group (2010). White Paper, *Self-Care: An Ethical Imperative*, SCCG, UK.

Thomas, K.J., Nicholl, J.P., and Coleman, P. (2001). Use and expenditure on complementary medicine in England: A population based study, *Complementary Therapies in Medicine*, **9(1)**, 2–11.

Tovey, P. and Adams, J. (2001). Primary care as intersecting social worlds, *Social Science and Medicine*, **52**, 695–706.

Wanless, D. (2002). *Securing our Future Health: Taking a Long-Term View*, Chancellor of the Exchequer's Review of Health Trends and Resources. Available at: http://www.hm-treasury.gov.uk/d/foi_dis_010205_wanless_ BUPA.pdf [Accessed Nov 2011].

White, T. (2010). *A Guide to the NHS*, Radcliffe Publishing, Oxford.

CHAPTER 9

Exploring a Model of Integrative Medicine: A Case Study in Swedish Primary Health Care

Tobias Sundberg

9.1 Introduction

This chapter provides a brief overview and research summary of a Swedish primary health care project developing, implementing and evaluating a model for integrative medicine (IM) in the management of low back pain (LBP) and neck pain (NP).

9.1.1 *Background*

IM is an emerging area in clinical health care delivery, medical education and research that generally targets an evidence-based approach to the integration of conventional medicine and complementary therapies (CTs) (National Center for Complementary and Alternative Medicine, 2010). IM expands on multiple concepts and frameworks in medicine, and approaches to integration may not only relate to the merging of different clinical perspectives and professional specialties, but may also involve different political, theoretical and philosophical aspects (Adams *et al.*, 2009). The great diversity of CT, modes of health care delivery and the degree of legitimacy and acceptance (or lack thereof) that CTs are afforded in various national policies, reveal the lack of commonly accepted working definitions and terms as well as the lack of official policies on how various CTs might be applied or integrated in the management of common medical conditions (Boon *et al.*, 2004; Cohen *et al.*, 2005; World Health Organization, 2003; 2005). Similarly, the clinical evidence base for comprehensive IM models integrating multiple professional, cultural and philosophical aspects of health and healing in conventional care settings is lacking, especially with regards to results from relevant pragmatic randomised clinical trials (RCTs).

9.1.2 *Aim and objectives*

The general aim of the IM research project was to explore the relevance of IM as a health service option in Swedish primary health care. The specific study objectives relevant to the focus of the current chapter are: Study I — to develop a consensus-based IM model adapted to Swedish primary health care and adhering to multiple stakeholders' perspectives including researchers, conventional care and CT providers; and Study II — to investigate the feasibility of implementing and testing the IM model's comparative effectiveness versus conventional primary health care in the management of patients with subacute to chronic non-specific LBP/NP. For other details of the wider study and results please see Sundberg *et al.* (2007; 2009).

9.2 Methodological Strategy

The general methodological strategy of the IM research project was to design research to gain a broad understanding of IM in the Swedish primary health care setting. Accordingly, acknowledging IM as a complex health care intervention (Campbell *et al.*, 2000; Walach *et al.*, 2006; Ritenbaugh *et al.*, 2003; Boon *et al.*, 2004), both qualitative and quantitative approaches were employed. In brief, the mix of study designs was combined in the following way: a qualitative health system research approach was used to develop the IM model (Study I). The IM model was then implemented and tested compared with conventional primary care in the management of patients with subacute to chronic non-specific LBP/NP, using a pragmatic pilot randomised clinical trial (RCT) with quantitative outcome measures (Study II). Notably, this way of combining qualitative and quantitative research methodologies, often known as triangulation, has been suggested to generate broader evidence-based knowledge on the use of CTs and other interventions in clinical health care compared with research strategies using a single methodological approach (Polit and Hungler, 1999; Walach *et al.*, 2006).

9.2.1 *Study I*

The development of the IM model in Study I was a highly clinical process (Sundberg *et al.*, 2007). A qualitative study design (Polit and Hungler, 1999) with an action research approach (White and Verhoef, 2005; Meyer, 2000) was used to develop the IM model on site in the clinical setting of a Swedish primary health care unit. Through multiple cycles of clinical group meetings and discussions with various stakeholders, the research group tried to gather increasingly focused information in order to exclude certain working possibilities and include others (Figure 9.1).

The IM model was developed through a number of key processes, i.e., research group activities, including regular meetings and educational seminars, snowballing for providers, deciding a target group and diagnostic criteria for patients, assessment of conventional and CT documentation procedures, the development of a project-specific documentation

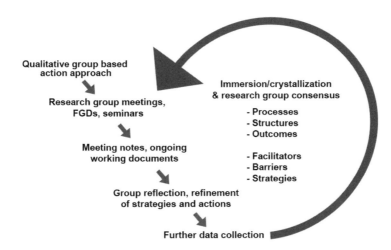

Fig. 9.1   An outline of the qualitative procedures and analyses developing the IM model (Sundberg *et al.*, 2007).

system with detailed IM patient records, testing and modifying logistical procedures including external and internal referrals and report mechanisms in relation to the inclusion and discharge of patients, and the identification of clinical outcome measures. As part of these processes, different stakeholders' perceptions and experiences relating to the integration of conventional care and CTs were discussed at the levels of patient/provider and the Swedish health system. A public health science framework which specified processes, structures and outcomes of the IM model was used to guide this approach (Donabedian, 1980; Handler *et al.*, 2001). Perceived facilitators, barriers and strategies for IM model development and implementation were discussed to aid clinical interpretation and applicability to the Swedish primary health care setting. The analytical process was based on the principles of immersion/ crystallisation (Borkan, 1999; Miller and Crabtree, 1994) and research group consensus (Boon *et al.*, 2004). Immersion/crystallisation is a methodological strategy suitable for clinical primary health care research which entails repetitive cycles of data collection, analysis, reflection and refinement of strategies and actions, followed by further data collection (Borkan, 1999; Miller and Crabtree, 1994). A consensus approach, arrived at by means of participatory input from the research group was considered essential, as the IM model aimed for integration rather than parallel practice of conventional and CT care (Boon *et al.*, 2004).

9.2.2 *Study II*

The pilot RCT in Study II (Sundberg *et al.*, 2009) used the reliable and valid SF-36 questionnaire, targeting eight health-related, quality-of-life domains (physical functioning, role-physical, bodily pain, general health, vitality, social functioning, role-emotional and mental health) (Persson *et al.*, 1998; Sullivan and Karlsson, 1998; Sullivan *et al.*, 1995), as the main outcome measure to investigate the feasibility and comparative effectiveness of the IM model versus conventional primary health care management for patients with subacute to chronic non-specific LBP/NP. Based on input from the IM research group, a set of clinically derived, but not scientifically validated, project-specific "IM-tailored outcomes" were used as secondary exploratory outcomes. These targeted: self-reported disability, stress, well-being (0–10 numerical rating scales), days in pain and the use of prescription and non-prescription analgesics, conventional care and CT (outside the IM model). The outcome changes between baseline and follow-up (a duration of four months) were used to explore and compare the results between the IM and conventional care groups using standard parametric and non-parametric statistical procedures. All patients were kept in their assigned groups. Patients lost to follow-up, i.e., observations with missing data, were excluded from the primary analyses. To comply with a more comprehensive intention-to-treat strategy, a secondary analysis was performed where the last observed measures were imputed for missing data. A significance level of 5% was employed and 95% confidence intervals were reported. All *p*-value calculations were two-tailed.

9.3 Results

9.3.1 *Study I — The IM model*

The aim of the first study was to develop a consensus-based IM model adapted to Swedish primary health care which adhered to multiple stakeholders' perspectives, including researchers, conventional care and CT providers. In order to address this aim the research utilised an IM model outcome which was characterised by a team-based integrative care process, intended to deliver a patient-centred mix of conventional and complementary medical solutions to facilitate the management of patients with non-specific LBP/NP of duration of at least two weeks (Sundberg *et al.*, 2007).

An important structure of the IM model was the establishment of the IM team — a general practitioner (GP) with knowledge of CTs and eight experienced CT providers with basic training in biomedicine representing the fields of Swedish massage therapy, manipulative therapy/naprapathy, shiatsu, acupuncture and qigong (both individual CTs and group-based self-help services were considered important in representing complementary aspects of care in the IM model). The integrative care was physically delivered using the structure of a conventional primary health care unit and a decentralised network of external CT practices. This was supported by a referral network structure of general practitioners from four neighbouring primary health care units. External funding was another structure that enabled CT patient fees to be set at a comfortable level in relation to conventional primary care fees (Sundberg *et al.*, 2007).

Adhering to the Stockholm county council's clinical practice guidelines (Stockholms Läns Landsting, 2009), the GP of the IM team was assigned a gatekeeping role with overall medical responsibility for patients. The GP's clinical role was to administer conventional care treatment plans and to discuss the appropriateness of integrating selected CT in dialogue with the patients and the IM team. Cases where CTs were to be integrated into the treatment plans (during the IM research project this was decided by randomisation) were then discussed every two to three weeks in clinical consensus case conferences with the entire IM provider team (Sundberg *et al.*, 2007).

During the consensus conferences the GP introduced a new case to the other team members by means of a presentation of the initial medical consultation with the patient and the set up of the conventional care treatment plan. The other team members then provided their input and through the consensus case discussions which followed, the IM team collaboratively identified treatment strategies tailored to the individual patient's ongoing needs and concerns. The patients participated in the health care process through personal interaction with the GP and the providers of CT during consultations. The IM management had a limit of 12 weeks and ten CT treatment sessions for each patient during the research project. Figure 9.2 describes the IM model and the care process in the individual case management of patients with LBP/NP.

Combining conventional and CT clinical reasoning with a non-hierarchical, open, continuous and parallel interchange of ideas through the consensus case conferences was positively experienced by the IM provider team, for example, in increased team-building and cross-fertilisation of ideas, leading to a perceived increase in diagnostic and therapeutic team capacities to verify and improve the ongoing clinical management of the patient (Sundberg *et al.*, 2007).

9.3.2 *Study II — The pilot RCT*

In the second study, the aim was to investigate the feasibility of implementing and testing the IM model's comparative clinical effectiveness

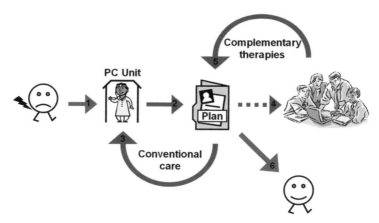

Fig. 9.2 The IM model and the IM care process illustrated as a clinical case management flowchart: (1) The patient with subacute to chronic non-specific LBP/NP consults the gatekeeping general practitioner at the primary care unit, (2) The general practitioner develops a conventional care treatment plan in dialogue with the patient, (3) The patient goes through the conventional care process, i.e., "treatment as usual", (4) Should CTs be considered appropriate, these are integrated into the treatment plan by way of a consensus case conference with the IM provider team, (5) The patient receives CTs as an integrated part of the treatment plan, i.e., the integrative care process is initiated, (6) When the treatment plan is completed the case management is finished. Please note that for the current research project the patients were assigned by randomisation and integrative care was only delivered for up to 12 weeks. PC Unit = primary care unit (Sundberg *et al.*, 2007).

versus conventional primary health care in the management of patients with subacute to chronic non-specific LBP/NP via a pragmatic pilot RCT. Of specific interest were patient and care characteristics, recruitment and retention rates, clinical differences and effect sizes between groups, and calculation of the adequate sample size for a full-scale trial supported by selected outcome measures and collected data (Sundberg *et al.*, 2009).

Seventy-five per cent (80/107) of patients seeking help for LBP/NP at the participating primary health care units during the IM research project were eligible and feasible for inclusion in the pilot RCT. Baseline characteristics of the 80 study participants by randomised groups showed that most patients were women (72–73%), in their forties, and more often had LBP (52–53%) than NP (33–36%). There were no statistically significant differences between the IM and conventional care groups at baseline (Sundberg *et al.*, 2009).

The characteristics of care identified that conventional management mainly included advice (85%) complemented by a prescription of analgesics (50%). Less-used GP strategies were sick leave (33%) and written physiotherapy referrals (26%). The IM model typically integrated two different types of CT into the conventional management. Swedish massage was the most common type of therapy to be combined with other types of CT. Shiatsu and qigong were the two most common CTs to be combined together. Manipulative therapy was the most common CT to be integrated as a single add-on treatment to conventional care. There were no reports of crucial adverse events with either conventional or integrative care (Sundberg *et al.*, 2009).

Approximately 80% of the patients completed follow-up after four months. In general, the outcome effect size analyses outlined large response variability with both types of care being equally as effective with no statistically significant differences between groups. A secondary analysis where the last observed measures were imputed for missing data did not produce changes to the results and there was a lack of statistically significant differences between the groups (Sundberg *et al.*, 2009).

Vitality was the only domain of the main outcome measure (SF-36, score 0–100) supported by both a clinically relevant difference between groups (Sullivan *et al.*, 2002; Sundberg *et al.*, 2007) and a small to moderate distribution-based effect size (Revicki *et al.*, 2006), i.e., -7.27 points (Cohen's *d* -0.34), which was in favour of IM (Sundberg *et al.*, 2009). Secondary outcomes in terms of self-rated disability and stress returned small clinical differences (0.66 and 1.18 points) and small effect sizes (Cohen's *d* 0.23 and 0.43) between groups supporting IM. Analysis of the use of health care resources showed a clinical trend between groups, with IM contributing to less use of prescription and non-prescription analgesics (-11.7 and -9.7% units respectively) compared with conventional care (Sundberg *et al.*, 2009).

Sample size calculations for SF-36 (vitality) with 80% power, 5% significance, a ten points clinical difference in change over time between groups (Sullivan *et al.*, 2002; Sundberg *et al.*, 2007) and the standard deviations derived from the pilot trial data, demonstrated the need for a minimum of 60 patients per arm to adequately power a future large-scale trial (Sundberg *et al.*, 2009).

9.4 Discussion

9.4.1 *Methodological strategy*

IM aims to contribute to a health care approach that is something greater than the mere sum of its parts (Bell *et al.*, 2002). In a similar way, a synthesis of evidence is increasingly enforced by health technology assessment boards to make informed decisions about evidence-based health care (National Institute for Health and Clinical Excellence, 2010; Rawlins, 2008). This research project embraced the concept of synthesis by applying a mixed methods approach to evaluation whereby the integration of different study designs, data collection methods and evaluation strategies contributed to a comprehensive framework to explore IM for LBP/NP in Swedish primary health care.

Several reasons and advantages of using a mixed methods approach have been proposed. For example, the use of mixed methods by definition contributes to overcoming the weaknesses of using any one method in isolation in order to understand a complex phenomenon (Polit and Hungler, 1999). This is commonly known as a complementarity of designs and methods. In the current project there were four main studies with different principle designs reasoned to provide complementing perspectives. First, a health services research approach based on a qualitative iterative group-based process was used to develop the IM model (Study I). This was followed by a pilot RCT with quantitative outcome measures to implement and test the comparative effectiveness of the developed IM model versus conventional primary health care (Study II). Third, a qualitative inquiry involving focus group discussions with patients from the RCT was conducted to explore experiences and perception regarding conventional and complementary care in order to generate possible care characteristics of IM (Study III) (Andersson *et al.*, 2012). Last, a health economic evaluation was performed to investigate the likelihood of IM being a cost-effective health service option in Swedish primary health care (Study IV).

Population-based surveys of CT utilisation have shown users to be predominantly well educated and from middle/high income groups (Hanssen *et al.*, 2005; Stockholms Läns Landsting, 2001). However, the geographical area purposively selected for the IM implementation in our study was largely characterised by higher rates of unemployment, lower incomes, more sick leave and more welfare support compared with the average levels in Stockholm at the time of the project (Stockholms Stads Utrednings- och Statistikkontor, 2006). Accordingly, the generalisation of the findings in relation to external validity (i.e., the relevance of the proposed IM model to other suburban primary care settings) in general or other low income contexts specifically, is believed to be high. Additionally, for solidarity and health equity reasons this approach was an important aspect of the IM research project.

The "black box" characteristics of the IM trial, where different intervention components may be identified but their contribution to the general effectiveness of the care in terms of specific efficacy cannot be quantified (Walach *et al.*, 2006), may challenge the possibility to reproduce consistent levels of intervention effectiveness in future studies. The interactive dialogues and decision-making processes of the IM team may also be difficult to standardise, which may contribute to large variability between different IM teams. Nonetheless, the recruitment process of patients through the primary care units, rather than via advertising in the media, is an important aspect which may serve to improve the generalisation of implementing the IM model in future clinical studies (through addressing "regular" patients seeking conventional primary health care).

The current results with generally small clinical differences and effect sizes between groups may challenge the use of a narrow set of outcomes measured in isolation to attempt to understand the relevance of IM in primary health care. The findings may further attest to the need of identifying additional relevant evaluation strategies, as suggested by recent outcomes research targeting IM and complex health interventions (Paterson *et al.*, 2009). The trend of decreased use of analgesics for IM in this pilot trial may support the use of health care resources as one such important target area. More disease-specific instruments with valid psychometric properties, such as the Oswestry Low Back Pain Disability Questionnaire, the Quebec Back Pain Disability Scale, and the Roland-Morris Low Back Pain Disability Questionnaire (Rocchi *et al.*, 2005), may provide another relevant area not specifically targeted in this pilot project. Additionally, aspects of prevention, lifestyle changes and health promotion (Long, 2009), more patient-tailored outcomes such as the MYMOP (Paterson, 1996), and a focus on processes of personal transformation and empowerment (Boon *et al.*, 2004) may also be important considerations.

However, while acknowledging the potential shortcomings of different instruments *per se*, the current evaluation strategy of iterative cycles integrating and triangulating quantitative and qualitative methods might still be one of the best approaches towards exploring complex interventions such as IM in clinical care settings (Campbell *et al.*, 2000).

9.4.2 *Developing the IM model*

The developed IM model was characterised by the adoption of a team-based approach to delivering a patient-centred integration of conventional care and CT, facilitated through consensus case conferences for patients with subacute to chronic non-specific LBP/NP. In acknowledgment of the diversity in approaches to delivering CTs with conventional care, different stages of collaboration have been proposed (Boon *et al.*, 2004). Accordingly, the developed IM model may be described as an "integrative health care" service option where health care providers collaborate on equal, non-hierarchical terms in the clinical delivery of care to patients. The consensus adhered to in the IM project has been suggested to increase in importance the further a health care practice model moves towards integrative care (Boon *et al.*, 2004). Interestingly, it was rare for the IM team providers to have experienced interactive medical dialogues communicating about patients with conventional health care providers elsewhere; a lack of communication and dialogue have also been described as barriers to IM implementation (Barrett *et al.*, 2003; Caspi *et al.*, 2000). The fact that all providers of the IM team, despite different clinical and philosophical backgrounds and medical models, shared a basic knowledge of biomedicine and CTs, may indeed have contributed to the atmosphere of respect whereby practitioners shared views on the patient cases which emerged (Anderson, 1999).

The group-based consensus approach of the developed IM model was seen as having several potential advantages over parallel or referral models of IM described elsewhere (Boon *et al.*, 2004; Frenkel and Borkan, 2003; Paterson and Peacock, 1995). Hypothetically, such advantages might include providing an IM model with increased team-building and cross-fertilisation of ideas, which could lead to increased diagnostic and therapeutic capacities, increased safety cross-checking, decreased risk of negative treatment interactions, increased resource sharing, reduced length of treatment cycles, reduced number of primary health care revisits, and improvement of health care cost-effectiveness by reducing health care costs (including the cost of drugs). However, although the IM team experienced a positive trend in terms of the collaborative group management of patients, most comparative advantages of IM over conventional care are yet to be statistically con-firmed in future larger-scale trials.

9.4.3 *Implementing and evaluating the IM model*

The current research project may be unique in that it has investigated a comprehensive IM model compared with conventional care (i.e., treat-ment as usual) in the management of regular primary health care patients with LBP/NP by means of a mixed methods research approach: typically, primary health care research of the CTs employed in the IM model investigate these CTs in isolation (e.g., RCTs comparing massage or manipulative therapy versus usual care) (Cherkin *et al.*, 2011; Hoving *et al.*, 2006; Korthals-de Bos *et al.*, 2003). Some recent insights into the lack of mixed methods research in IM suggest that this may be due to a lack of resources, organisational culture and logistical challenges for IM clinics (Boon *et al.*, 2004).

However, a relevant example of an RCT attempting to implement and test a more comprehensive IM model employed a "choice model" for patients with acute LBP (Eisenberg, 2005). Here, the patient's individual choice, rather than a consensus approach of an IM team, provided the basis for delivery of CT (massage, chiropractic or acupuncture) in addi-tion to conventional care. Patients were randomly assigned to the "choice model" combined with conventional care, or conventional care alone. Follow-up of symptoms, functional status and satisfaction with care was performed after five weeks. Costs of medical care were assessed after 12 weeks. The study identified no clinically significant improvements in symptoms or functional status between groups, although the choice group was more satisfied with the care. The CT care resulted in added costs, which were expressed in US dollars rather than costs per quality adjusted life year (Eisenberg, 2005). It was reasoned that future research should focus on patients with longer pain duration. Incidentally, our study complements this trial by investigating patients with subacute to chronic LBP/NP. The current clinical findings indicate that patients with chronic LBP/NP may be a more suitable study population for IM interventions than acute pain patients, although the current pilot study was underpowered to be able to statistically verify clinical trends in data.

The outcome measures that displayed the largest clinical differences in the pilot RCT (Study II), albeit within small ranges, were SF-36 (vitality) and the decreased use of prescription and non-prescription analgesics — both were in favour of IM. Clearly, less use of prescription analgesics, if confirmed, would be an important clinical finding which could reduce reported negative side effects linked to prolonged use of such drugs (Tramer *et al.*, 2000; Hernandez-Diaz and Garcia-Rodriguez, 2001). Perhaps the IM model, due to the individualisation of back/neck pain management through integration of CTs, facilitated additional and more individual ways of supporting and empowering patients compared with existing possibilities within conventional care services today. However, the added CT treatments may have encouraged more intensive management (e.g., by means of treatments, provider encounters or patient engagements during the treatment process), which in turn by itself may help to explain the trend towards more positive results for IM identified for some of the variables. Importantly, this increased "attention" effect was intentionally part of the IM model and was accommodated in the pragmatic and exploratory approaches utilised to investigate differences between models of care.

Interestingly, the majority of patients with spinal pain will not receive an anatomical pathological diagnosis explaining the cause of their pain (Krismer and van Tulder, 2007). Hence, most end up with "non-specific" LBP/NP. It is easy to imagine a degree of frustration here on behalf of the patients since the pain can be very "specific", severe and disabling. Additionally, this may also be a challenge for many conventional providers more familiar with relying on the verification of causative pathology for determining suitable treatments and care processes. This may in part provide an insight into why LBP/NP are the two most common reasons for patient consults with CT providers (Barnes *et al.*, 2008; Sibbritt and Adams, 2010). This may be an intriguing fact and a strong incentive for investigating the integration of selected CTs with an emerging evidence base into conventional care management of patients with LBP/NP.

9.4.4 *Global health policy perspective*

Most CTs are derived from ancient traditional medicine (TM) therapies and systems. From a global health policy perspective it is interesting to note that the World Health Organization (WHO) has issued normative recommendations for the appropriate use of TM/CT/IM in national health systems (WHO, 2003; 2008). The first WHO global TM strategy (WHO, 2002) was in part a response to the fact that many people suffer from various chronic illnesses, for which there may be no conventional treatment readily available in many nations, and in recognition that TM/complementary and alternative medicines (CAM)/IM may have many positive features such as improving quality-of-life for such chronic illness sufferers.

The increases in global CT use (WHO, 2002) challenge national health policies across the globe to simultaneously prioritise patient safety and treatment efficacy, yet offer choices which promote patient ownership of health (Knox *et al.*, 2009). In response to these challenges, many countries have established, or are in the process of establishing, a national CT policy. Norway may serve as an example of a Member State which has recently changed its legal framework to promote dialogue and a narrowing between the CT and conventional medicine sectors to partly stimulate IM research and development (Carlsson and Falkenberg, 2007; Helseog Omsorgsdepartementet i Norge, 2003). Coincidentally, Norway has also established a national research and information centre for CT (The National Research Center in Complementary and Alternative Medicine, 2010), a strategy that is encouraged by the WHO towards providing "evidence-based information on the quality, safety, efficacy and cost-effectiveness of traditional therapies so as to provide guidance to Member States on the definition of products and procedures to be included in national directives and proposals on traditional-medicine policy as used in national health systems."

Health conditions such as LBP/NP impose huge costs in many societies, and may be extra troublesome in countries lacking access to advanced technological medical care including pharmaceuticals. As suggested by the WHO, the TM/CT/IM sectors may add important additional resources and relevant practices in the context of primary health care services, particularly in scarce, low-income settings provided that they are proven safe, effective and appropriately used (also see Hollenberg and Torri, Chapter Five). Here, experience and supportive evidence from IM health care services research and development may contribute to health sector reform, particularly for low-income and middle-income countries, by bridging the gap between ancient TM systems and therapies and modern medicine. It is likely that health economic analyses would be more favourable towards IM service provision in such countries given that CT professional labour costs are generally much lower compared with the costs of conventional GPs and health care services.

9.5 Conclusions

IM is an emerging area of relevance for providers of conventional and complementary care in Sweden. In general, it can be concluded that the identification of IM facilitators, barriers and strategies by the different stakeholders contributed to the feasible IM services implementation within Swedish primary health care. The developed IM model adhered to standard clinical practice procedures and involved active partnership between a gatekeeping GP and a team of certified/licensed CT providers (Swedish massage therapy, manipulative therapy/naprapathy, shiatsu, acupuncture and qigong) in a consensus case conference model of care. It was feasible to conduct a pragmatic RCT comparing the IM model with conventional primary care in the management of patients with LBP/NP of mostly chronic duration. Exploring clinically relevant differences and the use of SF-36 (vitality) as the basis for a main outcome measure showed that the sample sizes per arm would need to be at least 60 to adequately power a full-scale trial. Triangulation of the various results suggests that IM is at least as effective as conventional care, with potential clinical benefits including empowerment and reduced need for analgesics. However, the current research project was explorative in nature and based on pilot trial data, and therefore the results should be interpreted with some caution. The findings attest to the need to further investigate IM as a complex health care intervention and to continue to explore relevant combinations of outcomes to help understand the relevance of IM in primary health care (e.g., by including patient and provider perspectives, detailed use of drugs and health care resources, and health economic evaluations). To verify the relevance of IM in Swedish primary health care, future research should prioritise larger trials considering large variability, chronic pain duration, small to moderate effect sizes, costs and longer-term follow-ups while adopting a mixed methods approach considering both general and disease-specific outcomes.

Acknowledgements

My sincere thanks to Dr Torkel Falkenberg, Associate Professor and Research Group Leader at Karolinska Institutet and Head at IC — The Integrative Care Science Centre, for providing excellent research support during the IM project. Thanks also to all co-researchers, conventional and complementary health care providers and patients who took part in this research project. The following Swedish organisations contributed with funding for the IM research project: Insamlingsstiftelsen för forskning om manuella terapier (Foundation for manual therapy research), Ekhagastiftelsen (Ekhaga foundation), Svensk förening för vetenskaplig homeopati (Swedish association for scientific homeopathy) and Skandinaviska Kiropraktorhögskolan (Scandinavian college of chiropractic). This chapter contains excerpts from Dr Sundberg's PhD thesis (Sundberg, 2010) and two related research papers (Sundberg *et al.*, 2007, Sundberg *et al.*, 2009). Additional publications from the Swedish IM research project are pending and interested readers are welcome to contact the author for further information.

References

Adams, J., Hollenberg, D., Broom, A., and Lui, C. (2009). Contextualising integration: A critical social science approach to integrative health care, *Journal of Manipulative and Physiological Therapeutics*, **32(9)**, 792–798.

Anderson, R. (1999). A case study in integrative medicine: Alternative theories and the language of biomedicine, *Journal of Alternative and Complementary Medicine*, **5**, 165–173.

Andersson, S., Sundberg, T., Johansson, E., and Falkenberg, T. (2012). Patients' experiences and perceptions of integrative care for back and neck pain, *Alternative Therapies in Health and Medicine*, **18(3)**, 25–32.

Barnes, P.M., Bloom, B., and Nahin, R. (2008). *Complementary and Alternative Medicine Use Among Adults and Children: United States, 2007. National Health Statistics Reports 12*, National Center for Health Statistics, Hyattsville, MD.

Barrett, B., Marchand, L., Scheder, J., Plane, M.B., Maberry, R., Appelbaum, D., Rakel, D., and Rabago, D. (2003). Themes of holism, empowerment, access, and legitimacy define complementary, alternative, and integrative medicine in relation to conventional biomedicine, *Journal of Alternative and Complementary Medicine*, **9**, 937–947.

Bell, I.R., Caspi, O., Sschwartz, G.E., Grant, K.L., Gaudet, T.W., Rychener, D., Maizes, V., and Weil, A. (2002). Integrative medicine and systemic outcomes research: Issues in the emergence of a new model for primary health care, *Archives in Internal Medicine*, **162**, 133–140.

Boon, H., Verhoef, M., O'Hara, D., and Findlay, B. (2004). From parallel practice to integrative health care: A conceptual framework, *BMC Health Services Research*, **4**, 15.

Borkan, J. (1999). "Immersion/Crystallization", in Crabtree, B.F. and Miller, W.L. (eds.), *Doing Qualitative Research*, Sage Publications, Thousand Oaks, CA, pp. 120–131.

Campbell, M., Fitzpatrick, R., Haines, A., Kinmonth, A.L., Sandercock, P., Spiegelhalter, D., and Tyrer, P. (2000). Framework for design and evaluation of complex interventions to improve health, *British Medical Journal*, **321**, 694–696.

Carlsson, P. and Falkenberg, T. (2007). *Integrativ Vård: Med Knventionella, Alternativa Och Komplementära Metoder*, Gothia Förlag, Stockholm.

Caspi, O., Bell, I.R., Rychener, D., Gaudet, T.W., and Weil, A. (2000). The Tower of Babel: Communication and medicine: An essay on medical education and complementary-alternative medicine, *Archives of Internal Medicine*, **160**, 3193–3195.

Cherkin, D.C., Sherman, K.J., Kahn, J., Wellman, R., Cook, A.J., Johnson, E., Erro, J., Delaney, K., and Deyo, R.A. (2011). A comparison of the effects of

2 types of massage and usual care on chronic low back pain: A randomized, controlled trial, *Annals of Internal Medicine*, **155**, 1–9.

Cohen, M., Penman, S., Pirotta, M., and Da Costa, C. (2005). The integration of complementary therapies in Australian general practice: Results of a national survey, *Journal of Alternative and Complementary Medicine*, **11**, 995–1004.

Donabedian, A. (1980). *The Definition of Quality and Approaches to its Assessment*, Health Administration Press, School of Public Health, University of Michigan, Ann Arbor, MI.

Eisenberg, D.M. (2005). The Institute of Medicine report on complementary and alternative medicine in the United States-personal reflections on its content and implications, *Alternative Therapies in Health and Medicine*, **11**, 10–15.

Frenkel, M.A. and Borkan, J.M. (2003). An approach for integrating complementary-alternative medicine into primary care, *Family Practice*, **20**, 324–332.

Handler, A., Issel, M., and Turnock, B. (2001). A conceptual framework to measure performance of the public health system, *American Journal of Public Health*, **91**, 1235–1239.

Hanssen, B., Grimsgaard, S., Launso, L., Fonnebo, V., Falkenberg, T., and Rasmussen, N.K. (2005). Use of complementary and alternative medicine in the Scandinavian countries, *Scandinavian Journal of Primary Health Care*, **23**, 57–62.

Helse- og omsorgsdepartementet i Norge. (2003). *Alternativ behandlingsloven — albhl. Lov om alternativ behandling av sykdom mv.* Available at: http://www.lovdata.no/all/nl-20030627–064.html [Accessed Sept 2006].

Hernandez-Diaz, S. and Garcia-Rodriguez, L.A. (2001). Epidemiologic assessment of the safety of conventional nonsteroidal anti-inflammatory drugs, *American Journal of Medicine*, **110**, 20–27.

Hoving, J.L., De Vet, H.C., Koes, B.W., Mameren, H., Deville, W.L., Van Der Windt, D.A., Assendelft, W.J., Pool, J.J., Scholten, R.J., Korthals-De Bos, I.B., and Bouter, L.M. (2006). Manual therapy, physical therapy, or continued care by the general practitioner for patients with neck pain: Long-term results from a pragmatic randomized clinical trial, *Clinical Journal of Pain*, **22**, 370–377.

Knox, K.E., Fonnebo, V., and Falkenberg, T. (2009). Emerging complementary and alternative medicine policy initiatives and the need for dialogue, *Journal of Alternative and Complementary Medicine*, **15**, 959–962.

Korthals-de Bos, I.B., Hoving, J.L., Van Tulder, M.W., Rutten-Van Molken, M.P., Ader, H.J., De Vet, H.C., Koes, B.W., Vondeling, H., and Bouter, L.M. (2003). Cost effectiveness of physiotherapy, manual therapy, and general practitioner care for neck pain: Economic evaluation alongside a randomised controlled trial, *British Medical Journal*, **326**, 911.

Krismer, M. and Van Tulder, M. (2007). Strategies for prevention and management of musculoskeletal conditions. Low back pain (non-specific), *Best Practice and Research: Clinical Rheumatology*, **21**, 77–91.

Long, A.F. (2009). The potential of complementary and alternative medicine in promoting well-being and critical health literacy: A prospective, observational study of shiatsu, *BMC Complementary and Alternative Medicine*, **9**, 19.

Meyer, J. (2000). Qualitative research in health care. Using qualitative methods in health related action research, *British Medical Journal*, **320**, 178–181.

Miller, W.L. and Crabtree, B.F. (1994). Qualitative analysis: how to begin making sense, *Family Practice Research Journal*, **14**, 289–297.

NAFKAM. (2010). *Nasjonalt forskningssenter innen komplementaer og alternativ medisin*. Available at: http://www.nafkam.no [Accessed Jan 2010].

National Center for Complementary and Alternative Medicine. (2010). *What is complementary and alternative medicine (CAM)?* Available at: http://nccam. nih.gov/health/whatiscam [Accessed Jan 2010].

National Institute for Health and Clinical Excellence. (2010). *About NICE.* Available at: http://www.nice.org.uk/aboutnice/ [Accessed Jan 2010].

Paterson, C. (1996). Measuring outcomes in primary care: A patient generated measure, MYMOP, compared with the SF-36 health survey, *British Medical Journal*, **312**, 1016–1020.

Paterson, C. and Peacock, W. (1995). Complementary practitioners as part of the primary health care team: Evaluation of one model, *British Journal of General Practice*, **45**, 255–258.

Paterson, C., Baarts, C., Launso, L., and Verhoef, M. (2009). Evaluating complex health interventions: A critical analysis of the 'outcomes' concept, *BMC Complementary and Alternative Medicine*, **9**, 18.

Persson, L.O., Karlsson, J., Bengtsson, C., Steen, B., and Sullivan, M. (1998). The Swedish SF-36 Health Survey II. Evaluation of clinical validity: Results from population studies of elderly and women in Gothenborg, *Journal of Clinical Epidemiology*, **51**, 1095–1103.

Polit, D. and Hungler, B. (1999). *Nursing Research: Principles and Methods*, Lippincott, Williams & Wilkins, Philiadelphia.

Rawlins, M. (2008). De Testimonio: On the evidence for decisions about the use of therapeutic interventions, *Clinical Medicine*, **8**, 579–588.

Revicki, D.A., Cella, D., Hays, R.D., Sloan, J.A., Lenderking, W.R., and Aaronson, N.K. (2006). Responsiveness and minimal important differences for patient reported outcomes, *Health and Quality of Life Outcomes*, **4**, 70.

Ritenbaugh, C., Verhoef, M., Fleishman, S., Boon, H., and Leis, A. (2003). Whole systems research: A discipline for studying complementary and alternative medicine, *Alternative Therapies in Health and Medicine*, **9**, 32–36.

Rocchi, M.B., Sisti, D., Benedetti, P., Valentini, M., Bellagamba, S., and Federici, A. (2005). Critical comparison of nine different self-administered questionnaires for the evaluation of disability caused by low back pain, *Eura Medicophysica*, **41**, 275–281.

Sibbritt, D. and Adams, J. (2010). Back pain amongst 8,910 young Australian women: A longitudinal analysis of the use of conventional providers, complementary and alternative medicine (CAM) practitioners and self-prescribed CAM, *Clinical Rheumatology*, **29**, 25–32.

Stockholms Läns Landsting. (2001). *Stockholmare och den komplementära medicinen*. Available at: http://www.sll.se/Handlingar/MPB/MPB%203/2003/Sammantr%C3%A4de%202003-04-23/punkt03bil1.pdf [Accessed Jan 2010]

Stockholms Läns Landsting. (2009). *VISS — Vårdinformation StorStockholm, handläggning vid sjukdomar*. Available at: http://www.viss.nu [Accessed May 2005].

Stockholms stads utrednings-och statistikkontor. (2006). *Medborgarstatistik*. Available at: http://www.statistikomstockholm.se [Accessed Aug 2006].

Sullivan, M. and Karlsson, J. (1998). The Swedish SF-36 Health Survey III. Evaluation of criterion-based validity: Results from normative population, *Journal of Clinical Epidemiology*, **51**, 1105–1113.

Sullivan, M., Karlsson, J., and Taft, C. (2002). Appendix F. *SF-36 Hälsoenkät: Svensk Manual och Tolkningsguide, 2:a upplagan*, Sahgrenska University Hospital, Göteborg.

Sullivan, M., Karlsson, J., and Ware, J.E. (1995). The Swedish SF-36 Health Survey-I. Evaluation of data quality, scaling assumptions, reliability and construct validity across general populations in Sweden, *Social Science and Medicine*, **41**, 1349–1358.

Sundberg, T. (2010). Exploring Integrative Medicine for Back and Neck Pain, *Neurobiology*, *Care Sciences and Society*, Karolinska Institutet, Stockholm.

Sundberg, T., Halpin, J., Warenmark, A., and Falkenberg, T. (2007). Towards a model for integrative medicine in Swedish primary care, *BMC Health Services Research*, **7**, 107.

Sundberg, T., Petzold, M., Wandell, P., Ryden, A., and Falkenberg, T. (2009). Exploring integrative medicine for back and neck pain — A pragmatic randomised clinical pilot trial, *BMC Complementary and Alternative Medicine*, **9**, 33.

Tramer, M.R., Moore, R.A., Reynolds, D.J., and McQuay, H.J. (2000). Quantitative estimation of rare adverse events which follow a biological progression: A new model applied to chronic NSAID use, *Pain*, **85**, 169–182.

Walach, H., Falkenberg, T., Fonnebo, V., Lewith, G., and Jonas, W.B. (2006). Circular instead of hierarchical: Methodological principles for the evaluation of complex interventions, *BMC Medical Research Methodology*, **6**, 29.

White, M.A. and Verhoef, M.J. (2005). Toward a patient-centered approach: Incorporating principles of participatory action research into clinical studies, *Integrative Cancer Therapies*, **4**, 21–24.

WHO (2002). *WHO Traditional Medicine Strategy 2002–2005*, World Health Organization, Geneva.

WHO (2003). *56th World Health Assembly Resolution on Traditional Medicine. Document WHA56.31*, World Health Organization, Geneva.

WHO (2005). *National Policy on Traditional Medicine and Regulation of Herbal Medicines. Report of a WHO Global Survey*, World Health Organization, Geneva.

WHO (2008). *Beijing Declaration. WHO Congress on Traditional Medicine, Beijing, China, 8 November 2008*, World Health Organization, Beijing.

CHAPTER 10

Integration in Primary Health Care: A Focus upon Practice and Education and the Importance of a Critical Social Science Perspective

Jon Adams, Daniel Hollenberg, Alex Broom, Amie Steel,
David Sibbritt, and Chi-Wai Lui

10.1 Introduction

In this chapter we argue that the mainstream work and commentary around integrative health care *and* education has often lacked a critical social science perspective. We introduce the framework of a critical social science perspective and explain how this perspective could be applied to the study of integrative health care (IHC) and integrative health education (IHE). Initially, we outline the popular models of IHC and their limitations and explore a critical social science perspective relating to such IHC practice and models. In the latter half of this chapter attention is then turned to examining key issues around IHE with the aim of presenting both a critical discussion of the principal theoretical ideas as well as an overview of the state-of-play of complementary and alternative medicine (CAM) in medical education. We first turn our attention below to describing the main tenets of a critical social science perspective.

10.2 A Critical Social Science Perspective

A critical social science perspective is concerned with a contextual analysis of power, knowledge and critique. In sociology, power is conceived as a multidimensional concept (Lukes, 2005). Although power is often understood as the ability of an individual or a group to make a decision in a conflict situation, this is not the only way power is manifest in daily life. In reality, power can also be an ability of the individual/group to set the agenda so that potential conflicts are suppressed or excluded — an ability of "non-decision-making". However, as Lukes (2005) points out, there is also a third dimension of power that refers to the ability to influence people's wishes or thoughts and make them act against their own interest. This third dimension of power is ideological in nature. This analysis of power provides an important conceptual tool to the study of health and illness and IHC. It directs researchers to various forms or strategies of domination that are embedded in health care settings and between different professional groups. The processes of medical professionalisation as well as integration involve the use of closure or exclusive strategies aiming to limit or regulate the entering of competitors into the market (Freidson, 2001).

The picture becomes even more complicated when the role of knowledge enters the discussion. Recent sociological studies on medical science have highlighted the conditions under which knowledge is incorporated into existing power relations and the constitutive role of knowledge in the production of new modes of domination (Foucault, 1973; 1980). This focus on subtlety and intricacies of power, knowledge and strategies offers a new angle to examine professionalisation and integration (Broom, 2006). Drawing upon the tenets of a critical social science perspective, we now turn our attention to applying such a perspective to the issue of IHC and IHE.

10.3 Prevailing Approaches/Models of IHC in Primary Health Care and their Limitations

Over the last decade, many health service researchers and theorists have constructed models to identify core values which may allow integrative care to be accomplished (Sundberg *et al.*, 2007; Myklebust *et al.*, 2008; Boon *et al.*, 2004a). Such commentators have suggested that the construction of conceptual models may help in identifying possible patterns or forms of collaboration of conventional medicine and CAM in different health settings (Boon *et al.*, 2004a; 2004b) and these have often taken the form of continuum models (Boon *et al.*, 2004b).

In addition to constructing analytical models, other researchers have also identified a number of critical elements or factors dictating success and influencing the ability to create the perfect IHC environment. These include adequate marketing, solid referrals, appropriate staff, effective record and communication, cross-professional education, provider compensation arrangement, as well as a supportive organisational structure (Barrett, 2003; Mulkins *et al.*, 2005). Another leading approach of defining IHC is the complex systems approach, which advocates treating the phenomenon of health or illness as an emergent property of a complex and dynamic system (Bell *et al.*, 2002). Drawing heavily on the sciences of biology and ecological philosophy, this approach emphasises that the ideal IHC model is a particular service arrangement, which facilitates conventional and alternative practitioners working harmoniously and as mutually supporting partners for the improvement of patient health. The systems approach to IHC attempts to go beyond the limitation of traditional thinking by shifting the focus of health integration from the individual discipline/practitioner to the symbiotic exchange between and cooperation across different kinds of health professions and practices (Dacher, 1995).

Although these mainstream approaches to studying IHC provide a useful set of conceptual tools for practitioners to describe integrative practices, they have limited value in accounting for the dynamics of IHC practice in general practice/primary health care (PHC) settings (amongst other settings). First of all, the discussions on IHC models tend to downplay the tensions and contradictions inherent in different paradigms of medical or health care practice. By conceptualising IHC as a matter determined largely by interests of the practitioners or organisation, the mainstream discussions bypass the issue of incommensurability between knowledge paradigms (Hollis and Lukes, 1982) and assume the blending together of biomedicine and CAM modalities as unproblematic.

However, this does not appear to be the case in terms of practice reality. Different medical paradigms often embrace radically different ontologies or mechanisms of disease causation and treatment (Ranjan, 1998; Coulter, 2004). It is not uncommon that explanation or prescription of one medical paradigm is incompatible with the other, and it can be extremely difficult (if not impossible) to bring them together in practice.

The second drawback of the mainstream approach is that the IHC models proposed are ideal types that are necessarily static constructs and may diverge radically from how "integration" is actually implemented or carried out in everyday health care settings (Clegg, 2007). Although it is acknowledged that the purpose of an ideal type is to highlight aspects of the world that may be heuristically valuable, there appear to be serious challenges to comparing and appropriating such ideal types with the empirical reality of integration as identified by research.

In fact, empirical studies demonstrate that the actual practices of IHC are very complicated and seldom come near to the neat patterns prescribed by conceptual models. Patterns of service provision are fundamentally shaped by the power and available resources of different professional groups as well as the dominant ideology of health care policy (Hollenberg, 2006).

A related problem of the conception of different integrative practices as a continuum is that the framework offers no explanation as to why a particular form of integrative practice would arise or prevail in a specific setting and, further, assumes that "complete" integration is in fact entirely possible as a final stage. In reality, ideal type constructs which fail to take into consideration social and historical specificities of medical practice have limited value in accounting for the dynamics of IHC. This is why a critical social science perspective is crucial to providing a more rounded understanding of the development and future of IHC.

10.4 Examining IHC from a Critical Social Science Perspective

In thinking about IHC critically, it is important to consider what is actually occurring inter-professionally between biomedicine (general practice/PHC) and CAM at the grass-roots as well as wider sociohistorical contexts. Simplistic notions and models of integration suggest a coming together of practices and/or practitioners and a sense that there is more linearity to health care delivery across the modalities available. Yet, using a critical social science perspective and situating the development of IHC in wider sociopolitical parameters and in processes of struggles for professionalisation and legitimation, we can see that the evolution of IHC and the relationship between conventional and alternative medicine are far from smooth and linear.

Historical studies on CAM movements since the nineteenth century reveal that the path of development of medical practice and the boundaries between different health paradigms are shaped by class, ethnic and sex relations in the wider society (Saks, 2003), as well as by the strategies and resources marshalled by specific movement leaders (Kelner *et al.*, 2006). While it has been argued that the increased role of CAM in health care could be seen as contributing to the deprofessionalisation of biomedicine (resulting from reductions in the monopolisation of medical knowledge, autonomy in work performance and authority over clients (Gray, 2002; Haug, 1988)), this argument of the waning power of influence of the medical profession has been challenged by recent research and has been shown to be oversimplified, if not erroneous.

For instance, works of Mizrachi *et al.* (2005) on various clinical settings in Israel confirm the existence of a dual process of simultaneous acceptance and marginalisation of alternative practitioners in health care settings. Although small numbers of CAM practitioners were allowed to practise and some of their techniques were absorbed by biomedical practitioners, they were seldom accepted as regular staff members; and their marginal status was marked by the use of structural, symbolic and geographical cues in the clinical setting that helped redraw the borders between conventional medicine and CAM. Similarly, Hollenberg's study on IHC settings in Canada found concepts such as "widespread collaboration", "synergism", "trust" and the like which are commonly used in IHC discourse, were rarely actualised in health care settings. In addition, biomedical practitioners were found to enact strategies of exclusionary and demarcationary closure that restricted the role and activities of alternative health practitioners. These strategies ranged from the use of "esoteric knowledge", dominating patient charting, referrals and diagnostic tests, to regulating alternative practitioners to specific "spheres of competence". Although the clinics under study offered some form of IHC practice with interactions between biomedical and alternative practitioners, these modes of practice or interaction did not resemble the theory or ideal typical models.

IHC may in fact be seen as more about strategic co-option of certain CAM procedures and technologies than the coming together of CAM and biomedicine (Broom and Tovey, 2008). The provision of CAM practices in biomedical settings may arguably result in a muting of metaphysical overtones (like notions of energy fields, qi or chakras) in an attempt to increase their compatibility with the biomedical model (Singer and Fisher, 2007). In turn, this process has also been exacerbated by processes of professionalisation and, in particular, the establishment of qualifications, licensing and regulatory bodies (Saks, 1998). As critically reflective sociologists, based on the above observations, we do not believe we are theoretically reifying the marginalisation that is readily apparent in IHC (Coulter, 1991). Although there are attempts to implement a more diverse model of health care delivery in certain contexts, there are also evolutionary processes occurring which may work against integration and produce new forms of appropriation and marginalisation (Cant and Sharma, 1999).

Perhaps most significantly, attempts at integration are not flattening power dynamics between professional groups (i.e., CAM and conventional PHC practitioners). Rather, biomedical practitioners are adapting strategically to the "challenge" of integration, reconfiguring their status as medical elites within the plurality of providers available. It is through a critical social science perspective that such processes of marginalisation, negotiation and co-option can be identified, unpacked and potentially addressed in future discussion of IHC.

10.5 Prevailing Approaches/Models of IHE in Primary Health Care and their Limitations

The skill and knowledge base of practising general practitioners (GPs) in relation to CAM is generally limited (Pirotta *et al.*, 2010) and paradigmatic divergences between CAM and biomedicine can complicate patient-doctor discussions regarding what constitutes "effectivenesss", "evidence" and "risk" (Broom and Tovey, 2007b). As such, there remains an urgent need for some form of CAM education at an undergraduate level for medical students. Specifically, there is increasing awareness within the biomedical community that in order to produce multiskilled and reflexive doctors, medical education must, at least in part, incorporate elements of CAM practice within its training programmes (CAHCIM, 2004). While

CAM education in medical curricula is an important development amid recent changes, there has been little sociological or critical social science analysis to date on this topic. Much of the debate regarding educational integration has been conducted and led by those in the practice field and has tended to promote one of a number of partisan positions and failed to subject the issue to wider cultural and political analysis.

In response, we here provide an introductory framework for exploring and appraising the status of CAM in medical undergraduate education, provide a critical sociological engagement with CAM education in the medical curriculum (including an overview of key issues and developments on the international scene) and examine the need for critical sociological teaching within such integrative educational programmes. This teaching should be offered as a means to improve successful communications and facilitate potential collaboration across different medical paradigms, as well as to create better understanding and contextualise patient decision-making and motivations regarding CAM use for medical students.

10.6 CAM in Undergraduate Medical Education: An Overview

There have been sporadic attempts to educate medical students about CAM in most developed countries and surveys appear to suggest that CAM incorporation into the medical undergraduate curriculum is growing apace (Wetzel *et al.*, 2003). For example, Cook *et al.* (2007) piloted an online CAM course for medical students and residents in the US and found that as a result participants felt more comfortable discussing CAM with patients, recognised a greater role for CAM and knew better where to find information on CAM. Similarly, Owen and Lewith (2001) developed a special study module on CAM as part of the Southampton (UK) Medical School undergraduate curriculum. Focusing on homeopathy, chiropractic, osteopathy and acupuncture, the module explored different models of health care, encouraged students to question their own assumptions about illness, and examined the evidence base for CAM. According to the results of a follow-up questionnaire, while some students became more sceptical about CAM, many others reported that they had developed an increased interest in CAM as a result of completing the module.

While providing a breakthrough in the coverage of CAM in such programmes (that would have appeared unimaginable a few decades ago), these CAM teachings, in electives or other compartmentalised offerings, do nevertheless tend to marginalise the significance of CAM. Such teachings also help bolster a medical culture where CAM is considered more a fringe activity engaging only a select few within the profession rather than exploring the possibility of CAM providing a set of complementary core values which can guide and refine broader conventional medical education and PHC practice in the future. Indeed, CAM, and the wider values that it embraces, has long been promoted as one possible means by which conventional PHC may improve its effectiveness and relationship to patients and may be a necessary antidote to what are sometimes seen as the invasive and insensitive (and ultimately unpopular) procedures and approaches to patient care (Berman, 2001; Frenkel and Ben-Arye, 2001; Park, 2002; Pietroni, 1992; Weil, 2000).

Unfortunately, the vast majority of the integrative programmes developed to date have been focused upon those at postgraduate and professional levels (Maizes *et al.*, 2002) and of those pitched at undergraduate level, the bulk has been concentrated within Bachelor of Health Science and Bachelor of Arts curricula programmes (Burke *et al.*, 2004). Exceptions to these rules are, however, beginning to emerge — with a small number of medical colleges in the US moving towards educational initiatives whereby CAM is woven seamlessly throughout the preclinical, clinical and graduate medical curricula (Sierpina and Kreitzer, 2005; Wetzel *et al.*, 2003).

Despite all these advances and developments in recent years, there is still an acknowledgement that programmes to effectively educate large numbers of up-and-coming medical students about CAM are desperately needed (Cook *et al.*, 2007; Wetzel *et al.*, 2003) and it does seem that such integration is highly likely, perhaps inevitable, given the exponential rise of CAM over recent years. A more interesting and pertinent range of questions facing such integration revolves around the future nature of such developments: who will provide the CAM teaching? To what extent will CAM be incorporated? How will integrative teachings sit alongside other professional educational movements such as evidence-based medicine (Marcus, 2001; Sampson, 2001)? And, given the time-starved nature of the medical undergraduate curriculum, what will be the potential casualties of such educational integration (what will be omitted from the syllabus) (Wetzel *et al.*, 2003)?

Just as attitudes to CAM are constantly evolving in the wider population, so too are those of medical students. Over the last decade there has been some research, particularly in the US, on the perceptions of medical students and their educators about CAM. For example, in their study, Lie and Boker (2006) found that medical educators were likely to have more positive attitudes towards CAM than interns and students. However, they also found that medical student attitudes to CAM (and CAM use) remained stable and largely positive and did not deteriorate over the course of training (such as through exposure to negative attitudes to CAM or immersion in the biomedical model). In another US study, Chaterji *et al.* (2007) found that, of the 266 first- and second-year medical students surveyed, nearly all (91%) agreed that biomedicine could benefit from CAM ideas and methods, and significantly, greater than 85% agreed that knowledge about CAM was crucial for their future as a health professional. Three quarters also felt that CAM should be included in the medical curriculum. Clearly more research is needed within different sociocultural contexts, but in general, support for CAM among medical students seems surprisingly high.

There is also some empirical work to suggest support for CAM may not be uniform across all student groups. For example, gender may play a role in mediating students' tendencies to utilise or indeed support CAM practices and CAM education. In a study by Greenfield *et al.* (2006), female medical students were significantly more likely than males to feel CAM has an important role in health care — a pattern potentially linked to wider CAM usage in the female population (Adams *et al.*, 2003). This difference *increased* through their medical education. Female medical students gave a more positive rating than males to the use of five CAM modalities, and moreover, females were more positive than males about learning the theory and practice of CAM and about increasing CAM curriculum time. Just as preferences for CAM (and support for science) are differentiated in wider societal terms, so too, it seems, are attitudes and perspectives among medical students. Increased diversity in terms of culture and religion of students in medical training contexts will no doubt influence such patterns, with further research needed on the ways in which different types of students respond to CAM practices.

While limited, there is some other research available that examines clinicians' perspectives on CAM training in medical education. In the context of PHC, perspectives on the value and need for CAM education have been shown to be quite varied. In an Australian study by Pirotta *et al.* (2000), most GPs (93%) agreed that there should be some education on complementary therapies in core medical undergraduate curricula. However, in this same study, the doctors surveyed were divided about the relative importance of this education for students versus conventional training modules.

One general theme throughout the literature in this area is the broad consensus that effective doctor-patient discussion about CAM is crucial *and* that adequate training on the part of doctors regarding CAM is the only way to achieve this. As noted by Caspi *et al.* (2000), the current scarcity of thorough exposure of biomedical practitioners to the diversity of CAM therapies and their fundamental concepts *and* of students of CAM to biomedicine and its related sciences, is far from ideal.

10.7 A Critical Sociology within CAM Medical Education and Examining IHE from a Critical Social Science Perspective

10.7.1 *A critical sociology within CAM medical education*

As explored in this chapter earlier, critical social science (sociology) can help illuminate key social, cultural, professional and political issues relating to CAM in medical undergraduate education. In the discussion below we argue that CAM could and should also be an integral component of any such integrative teaching. While sociology has a firm place in any well-rounded medical education, it is particularly useful, given the explicitly temporal and cultural variation and fluidity of the border between the two medicines (Adams, 2001; 2004b; Tovey and Adams, 2001). Below, we highlight key issues and opportunities that the discipline of sociology holds for CAM teaching in medical undergraduate education.

10.7.1.1 *Epistemological and ontological issues related to CAM and biomedicine*

There are some key issues and barriers in the introduction of CAM to biomedical education. The first, and the one most engaged with by medical sociologists (Coulter, 2004), is the issue of therapeutic paradigms, and the seemingly divergent ontological and epistemological positions of CAM versus those espoused by the biomedical model of disease. Indeed, much of the debate in the sociological and biomedical literature over the last two or three decades in relation to CAM has centred on "models of care" and the supposedly divergent perspectives of CAM and biomedicine on such things as: the nature of disease, the importance of the individual in therapeutic effect, key mechanisms of action and so on. These divergences, as far as we can meaningfully typologise CAM and biomedicine, engender ontological and epistemological positionings that medical students *must* understand in order to develop critical awareness of therapeutic pluralism. Moreover, in addition to ideological divergence, there are key language differences in CAM (for example, meridians, chakras or energy fields) which do not fit with the lexicon of biomedicine as currently taught to medical students, although this is not the case in all CAM (for example, osteopathy and chiropractic have increasingly framed their practices through a biomedical lens). As such, a genuine understanding of, say, naturopathy and homeopathy, is very difficult to achieve due to divergent views of the body and disease (Caspi *et al.*, 2000). In order to bridge language barriers, teaching a critical approach to ideological framing is crucial.

So what are the key ontological and epistemological issues and how might we make sense of the differences in ideological approach between CAM and biomedicine? Ontology, in this context, refers to the study of the nature of reality and epistemology refers to the study of knowledge or how we get to know certain things. CAM practice and biomedicine, in some cases, pursue quite different approaches to the reality of disease (ontology) and prioritise different ways of creating knowledge about disease and the body (epistemology). The biomedical model (the broad therapeutic approach espoused within biomedicine) entails a *functionalist* approach to illness, with an emphasis on the body as an organism that can be treated symptomatically. The biomedical model constructs illness as a breakdown or dysfunction of a particular organ. Medicine (especially hospital based but also community based) is broadly mechanistic, with doctors viewing the body as a machine made of many parts, with the respective individual parts treated separately. This mechanistic approach, crucially, stresses the centrality of the doctor in the healing process. The doctor's intervention is active, and, in general, downplays the role of any psychological or metaphysical factors which may cause the disease or play a role in its natural evolution or treatment. The biomedical model is thus characterised as *materialistic* in its focus on the corporeal body, yet at the same time abstract in its removal of the body from the soul and from the person. It is important at this point to stress that this is a model of health care, not a description of the actual approach taken by biomedical practitioners. However, in saying this, the centrality of this model in biomedical training and organisational culture does strongly influence how doctors approach treatment and is key within the curricula of medical undergraduate programmes internationally.

Ontologically speaking, CAM practices tend to focus on disease as an issue of (im)balance and as a reflection of systemic (rather than organ-centred) pathologies. As such, the body is viewed in a holistic rather than compartmentalised manner, and disease is viewed as specific to the individual person and body rather than abstractable in any meaningful way. A key factor in many CAM practices is the therapeutic relationship and the importance of interpersonal elements within the therapeutic process. Conceptualised as "placebo" within biomedicine, interactional dynamics are viewed as core facets of the treatment process. Moreover, "disease" is often viewed as natural rather than pathological *per se*, and treatment aimed at "healing" rather than cure.

To integrate discussion of and debate about CAM into biomedical education, the examination of these ideological differences is a key point of departure. Providing a critical understanding of the embeddedness of "best practice" in ideological positioning is critical for giving doctors insight into why their patients may use CAM, and as a means of encouraging debate about the nature of disease, therapeutic effect and wider divisions in health care provision.

In saying this, we should emphasise that while these broad typologies are useful to a degree, they also tend to reify distinctions that can be blurred in practice. Thus, as pedagogical tools they can, if deployed simplistically, be regressive in attempts to enhance medical students' understandings of therapeutic practices. Biomedicine, for example, does not always present a simplistic, coherent and linear ideological front. In fact, in grass-roots clinical practice, individual practitioners and subspecialities can present (and employ) quite different approaches to disease and to the patient. There are, for example, biomedical clinicians (and specialities) which broadly maintain a self-defined, patient centred and holistic approach to patient care (for example, factions within palliative medicine and subgroups within general practice). Moreover, some CAM practitioners pursue a largely mechanistic and positivist approach to the treatment of disease. For example, while some within chiropractic market themselves as holistic, others are relatively mechanistic in their clinical approach. Likewise, while homeopathy is seen by many as a system of medicine that fundamentally contradicts and challenges a biomedical perspective, in certain circumstances it can be approached and employed in a less challenging, standardised, first-aid fashion (this has been identified as a style of homeopathy employed by general practitioners) (Adams, 2004b). Similarly, acupuncture is, in some cases, utilised as a technical skill rather than a system of healing, and is deployed with little ideology in clinical practice. As such, teaching medical students over-simplistic paradigmatic divergences is inaccurate, in terms of what occurs in clinical contexts, and furthermore, may function to reify such differences and overstate incommensurability. We are thus left with a difficult choice: to teach philosophical difference and further compartmentalise CAM and biomedicine, or to reflect on the irreconcilability of such typologies in practice. In all probability, a combination of both is the best solution, emphasising difference and conflict but also interplay and cross-over where appropriate.

Understanding the ideologies underpinning therapeutic modalities is a critical component of medical education. However, there is also a need to understand why patients are utilising CAM practices, why there are sometimes conflicts between CAM and biomedicine and why some biomedical practitioners/organisations are against CAM integration? It is here that work performed on the sociology of CAM can help medical students make sense of such questions.

10.7.1.2 *Theoretical approaches to CAM: Conceptualising patient engagement*

It can be difficult, from a biomedical (or medico-student) perspective, to understand the varying reasons why people may actually use or gain benefit from CAM. Sociologists have been fascinated by the rise in popularity of CAM despite resistance from biomedical organisations and many practitioners and a virtual absence of state funding. To provide some explanation, sociologists have been delving into the sociocultural factors influencing this recent proliferation of the non-biomedical therapeutics. This work has drawn on a range of theoretical traditions with numerous attempts to highlight: a societal shift to "postmodernity", processes of reflexive modernisation and the emergence of new forms of "selfhood", to help conceptualise and explain CAM popularity (for example, Siahpush, 1998; Sointu 2006). These conceptual arguments, and others, may be useful in providing medical students and educators with useful frameworks for understanding the recently increased popularity of CAM.

The postmodernisation thesis has been popular among some CAM sociologists as an explanation for the increased presence of CAM. Its proponents view CAM use as reflecting wider patterns related to the "postmodernisation" of social life (for example, Siahpush, 1998). In this context postmodernisation is broadly seen to denote an increased fragmentation of experience, consumerism, individualisation and aestheticisation of social life. In the context of health care, metanarratives (for example, the biomedical model) are subsumed by subjective individualised knowledge which inform social practices and identity work. CAM use, within this model, is viewed as a rejection of the metanarratives related to disease and the selection, and production, of individualised understandings of disease-and-treatment regimes. Implicit in such arguments is the increased prioritisation of lay knowledge of disease and, importantly, the rejection of the superiority of scientific knowledge and expertise.

Social theorisations of late modernity have also been drawn on in attempts to conceptualise patients' preferences for CAM (Low, 2004). Moving beyond the rather over-simplistic "fragmentation of experience" and "individualisation" themes implicit in the postmodernisation thesis, authors like Beck (1992) and Giddens (1991) have focused on increased reflexivity in modern societies, and the tendency of "consumers" to be more critical of expert knowledge. The result, it has been argued, is that people have become more sceptical of the judgements or advice of (scientific) experts (Lupton and Tulloch, 2002), actively assessing the merits of particular claims. This in turn, it has been postulated, has opened up the potential for the proliferation of CAM — a backlash against the perceived failings of science and biomedical technologies (Kaptchuk and Eisenberg, 1998).

There have also been some recent attempts to theorise the potential implications, at an individual level, of new therapeutic models of care and their implications for changing notions of selfhood (for example, Doel and Segrott, 2003; Sointu, 2006). This work has examined the degree to which CAM use represents a significant shift in conceptions of disease and selfhood. In particular, the notion of well-being has emerged recently as a potentially useful concept for characterising what CAM offers the individual. Departing from biomedical notions of being "cured", "healthy" or "disease-free", well-being encapsulates notions of authenticity, recognition and self-determination, restructuring "health" as a subjective and individualised process (Bishop and Yardley, 2004; Sointu, 2006). CAM use is thus conceptualised as a project of the self — an individual search for recognition as being an authentic self that is both "discovered" by the individual and shaped by the nature of individual therapeutic practices.

Broom and Tovey (2007a) argue that while these theoretical ideas have some merit, what characterises patients' engagement with CAM is a complex dialectical tension between the appeal of individualisation and depersonalisation. Alternative models of healing, they argue, are valued, primarily, for their subjectified (rather than abstracted) and individualised (rather than depersonalised) approach — an approach seen to allow for and promote agency, self-determination and, ultimately, hope (Broom and Tovey, 2007b). CAM practitioners, they argue, promote a "project of the self" — a reclaiming of hope, subjectively and control — elements which were largely perceived to be neglected in biomedical care.

As sociologists, we argue for a critical, distanced approach to teaching about CAM in biomedical education. This involves teaching about the benefits *and* limitations of both CAM and biomedical models of care. Not all writing on CAM has focused on the positive liberating elements of non-biomedical therapeutics. Moreover, teaching about CAM will benefit

from a critical examination of how CAM-derived models of care may
have limitations for some patients with certain disease trajectories.

10.7.1.3 Theoretical approaches to the potential limitations of self-healing and self-help

The potentially restrictive, disciplinary or digressive aspects of CAM
therapeutics have received some attention in the biomedical and psychotherapeutic literature, where there has been some discussion of the potentially pathological discursive deployment of notions of self-healing and
self-responsibility on CAM therapeutic models. Permeating some CAM
practices are discourses of positivity and self-responsibility, engendering
quasi-metaphysical notions of self-actualisation and self-healing. What is
interesting, as sociologists, is the degree to which CAM-related ideological and rhetorical devices contain and deploy potentially restrictive (or
even spurious) models of therapeutic process. There is, as mentioned
above, an emerging critique within the psychotherapeutic literature
regarding the promotion of pseudo-spiritual ideas of self-healing and self-
responsibility. In this literature the ideals engendered in some CAM
approaches have been critiqued as toxic to patients' psychological and
physical health.

While some CAM practices (and models of care) are clearly extremely
helpful to patients, there may also be certain problems endemic in new
discourses around self-help and (spiritually mediated) self-actualisation.
An example is the ontological view, evident in some CAM practices, that
one can actively shape or change one's reality and that to heal oneself
necessarily involves an active reconstructing of one's world view and view
of the self. Such therapeutic frameworks ultimately denote a degree of
self-responsibility for disease or disease progression, and place the burden
of "reconceptualisation of reality" squarely on the individual patient. It is
not posited here that such conceptions are indeed *prima facie* negative or
positive for patients. Rather, what it does point to is a repositioning of
responsibility (and potential guilt) for those who find this state impossible
to achieve or indeed maintain. Such criticisms of CAM-related models of
care should also be included in teaching about CAM in undergraduate
medical education. Specifically, such possibilities should be placed

alongside representations of CAM models of healing as potentially useful and liberating for patients.

10.7.1.4 *Theorising the relationship of CAM to biomedicine: Inter- and intra-professional issues*

There has been a lot of sociological work undertaken on the inter- and intra-professional boundary disputes between CAM and biomedicine, especially conventional general practice and PHC (for example, Adams, 2004a; Hirschkorn and Bourgeault, 2005; Mizrachi *et al.*, 2005; Tovey and Adams, 2001). Here an emphasis has been placed on the complex dominance/subordination of various therapeutic modalities, shifts over time in public deference to biomedicine and increasing support for non-biomedical therapeutics (Adams, 2004a). For example, the Social Worlds Theory (SWT) has been developed as a useful explanatory tool for understanding the dynamics between CAM and general practice and this sociological framework can act as a highly effective conceptual tool for clinicians/students (both conventional PHC and CAM) in their studies of CAM and wider social, cultural, professional and political contexts.

SWT is useful in the case of educational CAM integration because it allows medical students to locate and contextualise the behaviours, practices and motivations of different professional groups (none more than CAM and conventional general practice or PHC). The formalising of ideas regarding social worlds has largely been carried out by Strauss, building upon the work of the key thinkers from the early Chicago tradition (Strauss, 1993). Central to the approach is the idea that society is constituted by multiple social worlds which "both touch and interpenetrate" (Clarke, 1990, p. 19). What is crucial to the perspective, however, is the fluidity of these worlds: how they are formed and re-formed by social action and how their fragmentation and proliferation into numerous sub-worlds is an inevitable consequence of processes within and between groups. A social world will characteristically be dominated by one main activity, have sites for that activity, involve technologies of one form or another, and be structured around some form of organisation. In these terms we can begin to approach CAM as one medical or healing world (incorporating many subworlds modelled around modalities) and conventional medicine as another health care world (also made up of sub-worlds such as general practice, rural health care, nursing and others).

At the heart of the SWT approach is a focus upon communication and language (both within a world and between worlds). Medical worlds can be conceptualised as universes of language whereby world members sanction and legitimise the actions and expressions of others in their world. Similarly, each world can also be approached as a paradigm that promotes and embodies its own language code. In terms of CAM and the conventional medical worlds (of which medical undergraduate education is a central component) there is indeed often a perception of divergent key concepts and ways of expressing and understanding health, illness and healing. Also of importance here is the SWT concept of intersection — the process through which subworlds overlap with a consequent transmission of knowledge — recognised by Strauss as being crucial in contemporary society, and one which has clear application to CAM in medical undergraduate education. The incorporation of CAM into medical undergraduate education is itself a prime example of a process of intersection whereby two worlds are moving towards an overlap of shared territory. In this case, the intersecting features yet to be finalised relate to the nature and extent of such intersection. It appears from current trends that the intersection will be "weak" — some of the territory and practices of CAM may be incorporated into the medical curricula, but this will not necessarily encourage or permit direct involvement from CAM practitioners and educators. Instead, CAM integration will be piecemeal and potentially secured in terms comfortable for, and managed exclusively by, medical-world members. While we have only provided a brief overview of key features, SWT (with necessary refinements and revisions) can provide an effective tool for medical students to appreciate and anticipate the cartography of contemporary health care organisation and its influence upon both cross-practitioner communications and clinical dynamics with the patient.

10.7.1.5 *CAM and the deprofessionalisation of medicine*

Understanding the potential impacts of the emergence of CAM for biomedicine (and conventional PHC) as a form of profession and expertise could also shape a key element of CAM-related medical undergraduate education. Again, sociologists have focused on both the dominance of biomedicine (over say, CAM) and the potential threat of CAM to biomedical hegemony (Saks, 1994). Specifically, although the biomedical community has to a certain degree maintained much of its control over health care delivery, a perceived relative warning in the dominance and professional autonomy of biomedicine has driven some sociologists to reflect on whether previous conceptualisations of "medical power" and "medical dominance" are actually relevant to contemporary health care organisation (Broom, 2006). Such debates have been prompted by such things as: increased public scepticism towards scientific and technological development, lack of recent progress in biomedicine in the treatment and prevention of disease, increased public questioning of "expert" knowledge and increased use of CAM (for example, Calnan *et al.*, 2005). Structural processes occurring within medicine, such as increased managerialism, have also prompted questions regarding the relevance of previous conceptualisations of the dominance of biomedicine in contemporary health care contexts (Gray, 2002). Specifically, this has resulted in the development of theorisations of a so-called waning in medical power and autonomy including the deprofessionalisation and proletarianisation theses. Proletarianisation represents the process whereby organisational and managerial changes divest professionals of the control they have enjoyed over their work (McKinlay and Arches, 1985). Deprofessionalisation, in the context of the medical profession, is associated with a demystification of medical expertise and increasing lay scepticism about health professionals. However, there is emerging evidence that the idea of CAM as a threat may have a potentially deprofessionalising impact within medicine may be inaccurate, with processes of strategic enlistment and translation occurring at the intersections of CAM and biomedicine (see Broom, 2006). Thus, models espousing a linear, power-based theorisation of CAM and biomedicine may create the illusion of a waning in biomedical power and patient support for biomedical expertise. Moreover, there is potential for CAM integration to bolster biomedical legitimacy and expert status (Broom and Tovey, 2007b), rather than CAM merely be viewed as a threat. Similarly, we argue that in teaching about CAM and biomedicine, while conflict and division may enhance understanding, students may begin to appreciate the interplay and potential commensurability of CAM and biomedicine by learning about the complex intersections and alignments existing between them.

10.8 Conclusion

The practice and education of conventional medical practitioners (for PHC) regarding CAM is in its infancy and much work is needed before CAM can be included as a meaningful and useful element in PHC practice and undergraduate medical education. In an increasingly pluralistic health care context, medical students and practitioners must receive the necessary knowledge base to allow them to engage with patients about CAM. The integration of CAM into both medical education and practice is an essential step forward in providing society with doctors who have had the opportunity to develop critical perspectives of therapeutic models. Sociology, we argue, is well placed to bridge the gap between advocates of CAM and those supporting the biomedical model, providing a set of critical perspectives for students and practitioners to think about the nature of disease, the body and the subject in contemporary society.

References

Adams, J. (2001). Enhancing holism? General practitioners' explanations of their complementary practice, *Complementary Health Practice Review*, **6(3)**, 193–204.

Adams, J. (2004a). "Demarcating the medical/non-medical border: Occupational boundary-work within GPs' accounts of their integrative practice", in Tovey, P., Easthope, G., and Adams, J. (eds.), *The Mainstreaming of Complementary and Alternative Medicine: Studies in Social Context*, Routledge, London.

Adams, J. (2004b). Examining the sites of interface between CAM and conventional health care: Extending the sociological gaze, *Complementary Therapies in Medicine*, **12**, 69–70.

Adams, J., Sibbritt, D., Easthope, G., and Young, A. (2003). The profile of women who consult alternative health practitioners in Australia, *Medical Journal of Australia*, **179**, 297–300.

Barrett, B. (2003). Alternative, complementary, and conventional medicine: Is integration upon us? *Journal of Alternative and Complementary Medicine*, **9**, 417–427.

Beck, U. (1992). *Risk Society*, Sage, London.

Bell, I., Caspi, O., Schwartz, G., Grant, K., Gaudet, T., Rychener, D., Maizes, V., and Weil, A. (2002). Integrative medicine and systemic outcomes research: Issues in the emergence of a new model for primary health care, *Archives in Internal Medicine*, **162**, 133–140.

Berman, B. (2001). Complementary medicine and medical education, *British Medical Journal*, **322**, 121–122.

Bishop, F. and Yardley, L. (2004). Constructing agency in treatment decisions, *Health,* **8**, 465–482.

Boon, H., Verhoef, M., O'Hara, D., and Findlay, B. (2004a). From parallel to practice to integrative health care: A conceptual framework, *BMC Health Services Research*, **4**, 1–5.

Boon, H., Verhoef, M., O'Hara, D., Findlay, B., and Majid, N. (2004b). Integrative healthcare: Arriving at a working definition, *Alternative Therapies in Health and Medicine*, **10**, 48–56.

Broom, A. (2006). Reflections on the centrality of power in medical sociology: An empirical test and theoretical elaboration, *Health Sociology Review*, **15**, 496–505.

Broom, A. and Tovey, P. (2007a). The dialectical tension between individuation and depersonalisation in cancer patients' mediation of complementary, alternative and biomedical cancer treatments, *Sociology*, **41**, 1021–1039.

Broom, A. and Tovey, P. (2007b). Therapeutic pluralism? Evidence, power and legitimacy in UK cancer services, *Sociology of Health and Illness*, **29**, 551–569.

Broom, A. and Tovey, P. (2008). *Therapeutic Pluralism? Exploring the Experiences of Cancer Patients and Professionals*, Routledge, London.

Burke, A., Peper, E., Burrows, K., and Kline, B. (2004). Developing the complementary and alternative medicine education infrastructure: Baccalaureate programs in the United States, *Journal of Alternative and Complementary Medicine*, **10**, 1115–1121.

CAHCIM (Consortium of Academic Health Centers for Integrative Medicine) (2004). *Curriculum in Integrative Medicine: A Guide for Medical Educators*, CAHCIM, Minnesota.

Calnan, M., Montaner, D., and Horne, R. (2005). How acceptable are innovative health care technologies? *Social Science and Medicine*, **60**, 1937–1948.

Cant, S. and Sharma, U. (1999). *New Medical Pluralism? Alternative Medicine, Doctors, Patient and the State*, UCL Press, London.

Caspi, O., Bell, I., Rychener, D., Gaudet, T., and Weil, A. (2000). The tower of Babel: Communication and medicine, *Archives of Internal Medicine*, **160**, 3193–3195.

Chaterji, R., Tractenberg, R., Amri, H., Lumpkin, M., Amorosi, S., and Haramati, A. (2007). A large-sample survey of first- and second-year medical student attitudes toward complementary and alternative medicine in the curriculum and in practice, *Alternative Therapies in Health and Medicine*, **13**, 30–35.

Clarke, A. (1990). "A social worlds research adventure", in Cozzens, S. and Gieryn, T. (eds.), *Theories of Science in Society*, Indiana University Press, Bloomington.

Clegg, S. (2007). "Ideal type", in Ritzer, G. (ed.), *Blackwell Encyclopedia of Sociology*, Blackwell, Oxford.

Cook, D., Gelula, M., Lee, M., Bauer, B., Dupras, D., and Schwartz, A. (2007). A web-based course on complementary medicine for medical students and residents improves knowledge and changes attitudes, *Teaching and Learning in Medicine*, **19**, 230–238.

Coulter, I. (1991). Sociological studies of the role of the chiropractor: An exercise in ideological hegemony? *Journal of Manipulative and Physiological Therapeutics*, **14**, 51–58.

Coulter, I. (2004). "Integration and paradigm clash: The practical difficulties of integrative medicine", in Tovey, P., Easthope, G., and Adams, J. (eds.), *The Mainstreaming of Complementary and Alternative Medicine: Studies in Social Context*, Routledge, London.

Dacher, E.S. (1995). A systems theory approach to an expanded medical model: A challenge for biomedicine, *Journal of Alternative and Complementary Medicine*, **1**, 187–196.

Doel, M. and Segrott, J. (2003). Self, health and gender: Complementary and alternative medicine in the British mass media, *Gender, Place and Culture*, **10**, 131–144.

Foucault, M. (1973). *The Birth of the Clinic: An Archaeology of Medical Perception*, Routledge, London.

Foucault, M. (1980). *Power/Knowledge: Selected Interviews and Other Writings, 1972–1977,* Pantheon Books, New York.

Freidson, E. (2001). *Professionalism: The Third Logic,* The University of Chicago Press, Chicago.

Frenkel, M. and Ben-Arye, E. (2001). The growing need to teach about complementary and alternative medicine: Questions and challenges, *Academic Medicine,* **76**, 251–254.

Giddens, A. (1991). *Modernity and Self-Identity: Self and Society in the Late Modern Age,* Stanford University Press, Palo Alta, CA.

Gray, D. (2002). Deprofessionalising doctors? The independence of the British medical profession is under unprecedented attack, *British Medical Journal,* **324**, 627–629.

Greenfield, S., Brown, R., Dawlatly, S., Reynolds, J., Roberts, S., and Dawlatly, R. (2006). Gender differences among medical students in attitudes to learning about complementary and alternative medicine, *Complementary Therapies in Medicine,* **14**, 207–212.

Haug, M.R. (1988). A re-examination of the hypothesis of physician deprofessionalisation, *Milibank Quarterly,* **66**, 48–56.

Hirschkorn, K. and Bourgeault, I. (2005). Conceptualising mainstream health care providers' behaviours in relation to complementary and alternative medicine, *Social Science and Medicine,* **61**, 157–170.

Hollenberg, D. (2006). Uncharted ground: Patterns of professional interaction among complementary/alternative and biomedical practitioners in integrative health care settings, *Social Science and Medicine,* **62**, 731–744.

Hollis, M. and Lukes, S. (eds.) (1982). *Rationality and Relativism,* Blackwell, Oxford.

Kaptchuk, T. and Eisenberg, D. (1998). The persuasive appeal of alternative medicine, *Annals of Internal Medicine,* **129**, 1061–1065.

Kelner, M., Wellman, B., Welsh, S., and Boon, H. (2006). How far can complementary and alternative medicine go? The case of chiropractic and homeopathy, *Social Science and Medicine,* **63**, 2617–2627.

Lie, D. and Boker, J. (2006). Comparative survey of complementary and alternative medicine (CAM) attitudes, use and information-seeking behaviour among medical students, residents and faculty, *BMC Medical Education,* **9**, 58.

Low, J. (2004). Managing safety and risk, *Health,* **8**, 445–463.

Lukes, S. (2005). *Power: A Radical View,* Palgrave, London.

Lupton, D. and Tulloch, J. (2002). "Risk is part of your life": Risk epistemologies among a group of Australians, *Sociology*, **36**, 317–335.

Maizes, V., Scheider, C., Bell, I., and Weil, A. (2002). Integrative medical education: Development and implementation of a comprehensive curriculum at the University of Arizona, *Academic Medicine*, **77**, 851–860.

Marcus, D. (2001). How should alternative medicine be taught to medical students and physicians? *Academic Medicine*, **76**, 224–229.

McKinlay, J. and Arches, J. (1985). Towards the proletarianisation of physicians, *International Journal of Health Services*, **15**, 161–195.

Mizrachi, N., Shuval, J., and Gross, S. (2005). Boundary at work: Alternative medicine in biomedical settings, *Sociology of Health and Illness*, **27**, 20–43.

Mulkins, A., Eng, J., and Verhoef, M. (2005). Working towards a model of integrative health care: Critical elements for an effective team, *Complementary Therapies in Medicine*, **13**, 115–122.

Myklebust, M., Pradhan, E.K., and Gorenflo, D. (2008). An integrative medicine patient care model and evaluation of its outcomes: The University of Michigan experience, *Journal of Alternative and Complementary Medicine*, **14**, 821–826.

Owen, D. and Lewith, G. (2001). Complementary and alternative medicine (CAM) in the undergraduate medical curriculum: The Southampton experience, *Medical Education*, **35**, 73–77.

Park, C. (2002). Diversity, the individual and proof of efficacy: Complementary and alternative medicine in medical education, *American Journal of Public Health*, **92**, 1568–1572.

Pietroni, P. (1992). *The Greening of Medicine*, Victor Gollancz, London.

Pirotta, M., Cohen, M., Kotsirilos, V., and Farish, S. (2000). Complementary therapies: Have they become accepted in general practice? *Medical Journal of Australia*, **172**, 105–109.

Pirotta, M., Kotsirilos, V., Brown, J., Adams, J., Morgan, T., and Williamson, M. (2010). Complementary medicine in general practice — a national survey of GP attitudes and knowledge, *Australian Family Physician*, **39(12)**, 946–950.

Ranjan, R. (1998). Magic or logic: Can "alternative" medicine be scientifically integrated into modern medical practice? *Advances in Mind Body Medicine*, **14**, 43–73.

Saks, M. (1988). "Medicine and complementary medicine: Challenges and change", in Scrambler, G. and Higgs, P. (eds.), *Modernity, Medicine and Health*, Routledge, London.

Saks, M. (1994). "The alternatives to medicine", in Gabe, J., Keheller, K., and Williams, G. (eds.), *Challenging Medicine*, Routledge, London.

Saks, M. (2003). *Orthodox and Alternative Medicine: Politics, Professionalisation, and Health Care*, Continuum, London.

Sampson, W. (2001). The need for educational reform in teaching about alternative therapies, *Academic Medicine*, **76**, 248–250.

Siahpush, M. (1998). Postmodern values, dissatisfaction with conventional medicine and popularity of alternative therapies, *Journal of Sociology*, **34**, 58–70.

Sierpina, V. and Kreitzer, M. (2005). Innovations in integrative health care education, *Explore*, **1**, 140–141.

Singer, J. and Fisher, K. (2007). The impact of co-option on herbalism: A bifurcation in epistemology and practice, *Health Sociology Review*, **16**, 18–26.

Sointu, E. (2006). Recognition and the creation of wellbeing, *Sociology*, **40**, 493–510.

Strauss, A. (1993). *Continual Permutations of Action*, Aldine de Gruyter, New York.

Sundberg, T., Haplin, J., Warenmark, A., and Falkenberg, T. (2007). Towards a model for integrative medicine in Swedish primary care, *BMC Health Services Research*, **7**, 1–9.

Tovey, P. and Adams, J. (2001). Primary care as intersecting social worlds, *Social Science and Medicine*, **52**, 695–706.

Weil, A. (2000). The significance of integrative medicine for the future of medical education, *American Journal of Medicine*, **108**, 441–443.

Wetzel, M., Kaptchuk, T., Haramati, A., and Eisenberg, D. (2003). Complementary and alternative medical therapies: Implications for medical education, *Annals of Internal Medicine*, **138**, 191–196.

Index

acupuncture   1, 11, 53, 75, 95, 165,
    167, 175, 185, 192, 209, 215
Adams, Jon   1, 2, 4, 5, 7, 11, 12, 23,
    27, 39, 42, 43, 51, 57, 61, 62, 73,
    77–79, 81, 83, 93, 95, 96, 106, 115–
    117, 119, 123, 126, 149, 158, 160,
    181, 194, 203, 211, 212, 215, 219
Andrews, Gavin   40–42, 117, 121
Andrews, Jon   38, 40, 41
anthropology
    anthropological   104
    anthropologists   103
    anthroposophical   137, 140
aromatherapy   17, 19, 53, 122, 177
Ayurveda   17, 18, 74, 96, 100
    Ayurvedic therapies   53

Broom, Alex   11, 115, 203, 204,
    208, 217, 221

cancers   23, 26, 35, 73, 78, 79, 95
children   58, 59, 61, 82, 98, 144
Chinese medicine   17, 19, 74, 76, 93
chiropractic   1, 11, 23, 76, 93, 118,
    122, 192, 209, 213, 215
    chiropractors   17, 18, 22, 118,
        119, 123, 124

chronic illnesses   35, 37, 38, 40, 43,
    159, 161, 169, 194
Cramer, Helen   6, 133

dermatology   55, 56, 77
    dermatologist   142
dietary   58, 75
    dietary change   165
    dietary supplements   58
doctors   15, 17, 20, 21, 25, 38, 41,
    52, 77, 80, 117, 140, 142, 144,
    148, 157, 159, 160–162, 164, 166,
    168, 169, 208, 212, 214, 222

economic analysis/methods   195
    economic evaluations   189,
        196
    economic significance   100
ethics   5, 51
    ethical approval   16, 120
evidence-based approach   181
evidence-based health care
    189
evidence-based information   24
evidence-based knowledge   183
evidence-based medicine
    (EBM)   105, 166, 194, 210

evidence-based options   167
evidence-based scientific
   management   161

family physicians   37, 38, 117

Gavin, Andrews   35
general practice   1–7, 51, 55, 56,
   115, 117, 205, 215, 219, 220
general practitioners (GPs)   2,
   14–16, 21, 22, 24, 26, 27, 37, 51,
   59–62, 76, 115, 117, 119, 120–124,
   134, 141, 142, 148, 149, 158, 159,
   160, 161, 164, 165, 166, 167,
   185–188, 195, 208, 212, 215
geographical   189

health services research   126, 189
Hollenberg, Daniel   5, 93, 95–98,
   104, 105, 108, 203, 206, 207
homeopathy   53, 74–76, 93, 95, 140,
   143, 146, 176, 209, 213, 215

Lewith, George   209

massage   1, 22, 23, 39, 53, 59, 95,
   122, 176, 177, 185, 188, 192, 195
      massage therapists   18, 22, 39
meditation   17–19, 22, 23, 95, 122,
   165
menopause   11–15, 24, 26, 165
midwifery   95

National Center for Complementary
   and Alternative Medicine   181
naturopathy   1, 74–76, 78, 79, 83,
   86, 93, 95, 116, 118, 213
nursing   220

older people   35, 38–43, 116
osteopathy   11, 17, 18, 76, 116, 167,
   209, 213
      osteopath   17, 18

Peters, David   2, 4, 6, 157, 159
pharmacists   2, 15, 17, 19, 20,
   24–26,37, 133, 134, 136–138,
   144–147
pharmacy   6, 15, 26, 133–150
      poly-pharmacy   160
population aging   40
pregnancy   144
public health   79, 104, 107, 125,
   126, 168, 184

qualitative research   80, 98, 120,
   158, 182, 183, 189, 191

Randomized Controlled Trials
   (RCT)   105
reflexology   53, 144
regulation   81–85, 134, 168, 169
research capacity building   3
risks   5, 58–60, 62, 81, 82, 116, 126,
   159, 192, 208
rural health   5, 115, 117, 125, 126,
   220

Sibbritt, David   11, 39, 115, 123,
   194, 203
skin diseases   4, 5, 51–57, 60, 61
Steel, Amie   4, 11, 203
Sundberg, Tobias   6, 181–188, 196,
   204

t'ai chi   165
therapists   39